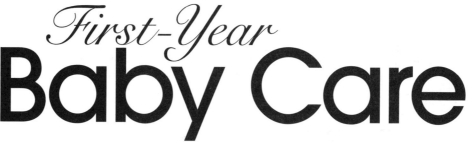

First-Year Baby Care

The "Owner's Manual" You Need for Your Baby's First Year

by Paula Kelly MD

Meadowbrook Press
Distributed by Simon & Schuster
New York

Library of Congress Cataloging-in-Publication Data

Names: Kelly, Paula, 1949- author.
Title: First-year baby care : an illustrated step-by-step guide / by Paula Kelly, MD.
Description: Minnetonka, Minnesota : Meadowbrook Press New York ; Distributed by Simon & Schuster, [2016] | Includes index.
Identifiers: LCCN 2015048201 (print) | LCCN 2016005934 (ebook) |
  ISBN 9781501112737 (S&S pbk.) | ISBN 9780881665734 (MBP pbk.) | ISBN 9781451669619 (ebook)
Subjects: LCSH: Infants--Care--Popular works. | Infants--Health and hygiene--Popular works.
Classification: LCC RJ61 .K324 2016 (print) | LCC RJ61 (ebook) | DDC 618.92/01--dc23
LC record available at http://lccn.loc.gov/2015048201

Medical Editor: Paula Kelly, MD
Copy Editor: Laura Silver
Creative Director: Tamara JM Peterson
Illustrations: Karen Martin, Patricia Carey, and Susan Spellman
Index: Beverlee Day
Cover Photo: JGI/Tom Grill

Thank you to Parent Trust for Washington Children for permission to reprint the material on baby exercises. Some of the material in the medical care section first appeared, in a slightly different form, in *The Parent's Guide to Baby and Child Medical Care*, edited by Terril H. Hart, MD (Meadowbrook, 1982).

Published by Meadowbrook Press
6110 Blue Circle Drive, Suite 237
Minnetonka, Minnesota 55343

www.meadowbrookpress.com

BOOK TRADE DISTRIBUTION by Simon and Schuster
a division of Simon and Schuster, Inc.
1230 Avenue of the Americas
New York, New York 10020

20 19 18 17 16   10 9 8 7 6 5 4 3 2

Printed in the United States of America

Contents

Introduction

Becoming a new parent is one of the most thrilling experiences you'll ever have; in fact, I often refer to the birth of a child as life's premier event. It's also one of the most challenging. *First-Year Baby Care* will guide you through your new parenting responsibilities when you'll likely need it most—during your baby's first year. This book provides you with much-needed encouragement and essential tips that will boost your skills and help you care for your baby with confidence and competence.

Today, many new parents spend little time in the hospital or birth center after their babies are born. They can't rely on the hospital or birth center staff to teach them all they'll need to know about caring for newborns. Newborn classes can provide important information, but many parents still find themselves wondering and worrying about how to keep their babies healthy and safe.

This book's goal is to help fill in the gaps. As a pediatrician, I've found that new parents often raise the same questions about baby care. They wonder about everyday matters, like how to bathe a baby or childproof a home, and more complicated ones, like finding day care, monitoring child development, and handling medical problems. As a brand-new first-time grandparent, I am especially motivated to make sure I am up to date on both the science and the art of parenting. By listening carefully to the concerns of new parents (including my own grown children), and by tapping into the wisdom of experts, I've put together everything you need for this first blissful yet daunting year.

This fifth edition builds on the practical, easy-to-follow information in the first four editions. In it you'll still find illustrated step-by-step instructions and essential facts on caring for and feeding your baby and keeping him safe and healthy, alongside the latest knowledge on a variety of parenting topics, from breastfeeding, sleeping, and introducing solid foods to choosing developmentally appropriate toys and traveling with your baby. We've added key facts on topics like nutrition and the sometimes contentious topic of vaccinations and prevention of disease and included new resources to help busy (and possibly bewildered) new parents manage their new roles.

Your baby's first year will test your resolve and give you many moments of great joy. I hope this book helps you rise to the challenges and appreciate the wonderful new addition to your family.

Paula Kelly

Paula Kelly, MD

P.S. In recognition of the fact that children do indeed come in both sexes, and in an effort to represent each, the use of masculine and feminine pronouns will alternate with each chapter.

Before Your Baby Arrives

You have lots to do before your baby is born—choose a name, decorate the nursery, buy supplies. The following tasks, however, may be the most important, because they'll benefit your baby's well-being—and yours—before and after he's born.

Take Care of Yourself

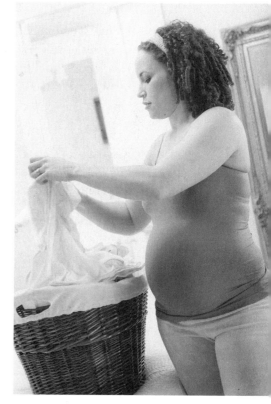

Birth defects are the leading cause of infant death. By taking care of yourself during pregnancy, you help prevent birth defects. Here's what you can do:

- Eat well. Try to eat the recommended number of servings from each of the five main food groups. Strive for variety in your diet. Drink at least ten 8-ounce glasses of fluid a day. You will need more when you are exercising or in a warm environment. The foods you eat fulfill some of your fluid intake needs, especially fruits and vegetables. Consume salt in moderation. Consult the latest dietary guidelines from the United States Department of Agriculture (http://www.nutrition.gov). Talk to your health care provider about taking a prenatal vitamin to make sure you're getting essential nutrients, minerals, and vitamins—especially calcium, iron, and folic acid (a B vitamin that helps decrease the incidence of spina bifida and other birth defects). You may want to increase your omega-3 fatty acid and vitamin D intake as well, to encourage optimum brain and eye development and build strong bones and teeth for your baby. Avoid consuming fish that are high in mercury, raw fish, saccharin, unpasteurized milk and cheese, and lunch meats, and talk to your care provider about other foods to limit or avoid. Reduce your caffeine intake.

- Have regular checkups, to assure you get the recommended prenatal blood tests and ultrasounds. Your care provider will follow your weight and blood pressure and screen for diabetes and, later in your pregnancy, the presence of Group B streptococcus (GBS) bacteria. GBS is the most common cause among newborns of blood and brain infections. Taking antibiotics before delivery can prevent transmission to your baby.

- Make sure your vaccinations are current, especially the rubella (German measles) vaccination. Acquiring an infection from this disease during early pregnancy can result in serious heart, vision, and hearing problems for your baby. A Tdap (tetanus, diphtheria, and whooping cough, also known as pertussis) vaccine is also recommended for every pregnant mother to get during the third trimester of every pregnancy. Whooping cough is a very serious infection for a young infant, and immunizing the mother will help give important protection.

- Alert your care provider to any illnesses you are exposed to during pregnancy, including fifth disease (parvovirus B19), chicken pox (varicella), and cytomegalovirus (CMV). Though uncommon, some illnesses can cause problems for your fetus.

- Exercise regularly. Talk to your care provider about what kinds of exercise are right for you and in what amounts.

- Avoid alcohol, cigarettes, and recreational drugs. These substances can affect your fetus's physical and emotional development. Also, talk to your care provider before taking any prescription medications.

- Avoid environmental hazards:
  - Avoid chemicals found in certain workplaces such as industrial plants and in some household cleaning products.
  - Don't drink water that contains high levels of lead or pesticides.
  - Avoid contact with litter boxes and rodent droppings. Both cat and rodent feces are linked to diseases (toxoplasmosis and lymphocytic choriomeningitis virus, respectively) that can cause birth defects, physical or mental delays, or miscarriage.
  - Avoid tanning booths completely.
  - There are some restrictions on hot tub use; please check with your care provider.
  - Many studies are being conducted to test radio waves and radiation emitted from Wi-Fi and mobile devices. So far the studies have been inconclusive, but erring on the side of caution might be a good idea. Continue to use your laptop, cell phone, and other mobile devices; just keep them away from your body when they are not in use.
  - Most importantly, always wear your seat belt.

- Assess your family history and your partner's for risk factors. A family health history questionnaire is available at the March of Dimes website (http://www.marchofdimes .com/pregnancy/trying_healthhistory.html).

Choose the Right Birth Place

When selecting your maternity care provider and birth place, ask plenty of questions about their policies and procedures. Knowing what to expect will help ease your mind and prepare you for the birth. Find out about their rooming-in policy. (Will it be possible for your baby to stay with you after the birth to bond and breastfeed?) A birth place with a "Baby-Friendly" designation has met criteria to support breastfeeding. (See https://www .babyfriendlyusa.org for a list of hospitals with this distinction.) Find out what expertise is available for emergency procedures. Although it's unlikely that something will go wrong, if you need an emergency cesarean or your baby arrives earlier than expected or ill, you'll want to know that your birth place has proper newborn resuscitation capabilities and appropriate nursery care for premature and sick babies. Be sure you're comfortable with your provider and birth place, so you and your baby get the best care possible.

Some parents list their goals and desires for the birth in a birth plan. Consider creating your own with consultation from your care provider.

Choose a Health Care Provider for Your Baby

Around the twenty-fourth week of your pregnancy, your own care provider will encourage you to select a health care provider for your baby. You'll spend a great deal of time at the care provider's office for well-child visits during the first year, so it's important that you trust, respect, and feel comfortable with him or her.

The following is a list of different types of pediatric care providers. Make sure the care provider you choose is covered by your insurance plan.

- Pediatrician—a doctor of medicine (MD) who specializes in children's health care
- Family physician—an MD who provides care for the entire family
- General practitioner—an MD or a doctor of osteopathy (DO) who can provide pediatric or family health care
- Pediatric or family nurse practitioner—a registered nurse with additional training and certification in pediatric or family health care
- Physician's assistant—a graduate of two-year training program in primary medicine who provides pediatric services under the supervision of a physician
- Naturopathic physician—a doctor of naturopathic medicine (ND) who provides well-child care, emphasizes the nonmedical treatment of illnesses, and refers seriously ill children to medical doctors
- Perinatologist—a specialist in newborn medicine who's needed when it's known though prenatal testing that a baby will have a birth defect or other special needs
- Neonatologist or a neonatal nurse practitioner—a medical specialist who cares for newborns (such as premature babies) who are sick or require nonroutine newborn care

You can find a care provider for your baby using the following resources:

- Your own primary care provider, if you intend to choose a different care provider for your child
- Birth center of a hospital or clinic, especially postpartum and nursery nursing staff: Nurses see the care providers at work with both mothers and babies and can therefore give you excellent advice and information.
- Health insurance provider directory: Your selection might be confined to a specific group of health care providers. Your health insurance provider may have an app to help you find a provider.

- Friends with children: Parents usually have strong feelings about their pediatric care providers. Consider both positive and negative comments.
- Online care provider locators, such as the American Academy of Pediatrics (AAP) Pediatrician Referral Service at http://www.aap.org, or Angie's List at http://www.angieslist.com
- County health association or board of health
- *The Official ABMS Directory of Board Certified Medical Specialists* (available at your local library or online at http://www.abmsdirectory.com)
- Local chapters of care provider associations, such as the AAP, AAFP, or the American Medical Association (AMA)
- Teaching hospitals
- Telephone directory Yellow Pages, under Physicians, Family Practice, or Pediatrics
- Local magazine listings of "Top Doctors"

It's important to interview your child's care provider. When choosing one, take into account your philosophy and approach to health care. Do you want to play an active role in your child's health care, or do you want to rely on the care provider's authority? Would you rather see a care provider who's in a solo, small group, or large clinic practice? Do you want to go to an office that just sees children or one that sees all ages? Do you prefer an office that does only primary care or one that also offers multispecialty care? What are your views on breastfeeding? Circumcision? Infant sleep? Once you've answered these kinds of questions, ask a potential care provider several questions about his or her:

- Training, experience, and affiliations (*When and where did you receive your medical training? Are you board certified?*)
- Medical philosophy (*How can I best help you to do your job caring for my baby? How do you view the parent's role in a child's health care?*)
- Standard schedule of care (*How soon after my baby's initial exam would you like to see him again?*)
- Availability (*When are you at the office? What is coverage when you are not at the clinic or the clinic is closed? Are you available by phone and/or e-mail?*)
- Office staff and resources (*What other professional staff are available at your office? What are their roles? To what hospital do you admit your patients?*)
- Office management (*How are well-child appointments scheduled? Do you have an online patient portal so I can have access to my baby's records?*)

Do the care provider's answers match your philosophy and approach to health care? If they don't, move on to the next potential care provider. If they do, double-check with parents of current and past patients. Are they satisfied with the care provider's quality of care? After considering all the information, trust your own feelings about a care provider. If you feel comfortable with him or her, your child likely will, too.

Decide Whether to Breastfeed or Formula Feed Your Baby

A slew of studies in recent years have shown how important breastfeeding is to the well-being of babies, mothers, and society. This has fueled a resurgence of breastfeeding in North America, which was a formula-feeding culture for several decades. Both options are open to you as a new mom.

It is best to decide well ahead of your delivery whether to breast or bottle feed your baby. Deciding before the birth gives you time to buy supplies (for example, breast pump or bottles) and, if you choose to breastfeed, arrange to take breastfeeding classes and build a breastfeeding support system.

Your baby should "room in" or stay with you as much as possible while you're at the hospital or birth center, but especially if you plan to breastfeed. The "Baby-Friendly" designation lets you know if your hospital is committed to keeping mom and baby together as much as possible. See https://www.babyfriendlyusa.org for a list of hospitals with this distinction. Make your breastfeeding plans and wishes very clear to the birthing staff before your baby is born.

Learn about Newborn Exams and Procedures

After the birth, a care provider will examine your newborn thoroughly and perform exams and tests to evaluate his well-being. (See page 13.) While these routine procedures are no cause for alarm and have been found to have important benefits, it may ease your mind to discuss any concerns or questions you have about them beforehand.

Decide about Circumcision

Circumcision is a surgical procedure that removes some of the skin that covers the tip of

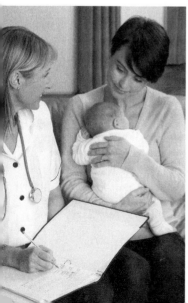

the penis (foreskin). Decide whether to have a baby boy circumcised well in advance of delivery. This procedure is performed by an experienced person (medical professional or religious officiant), and it usually happens before the baby leaves the hospital or birth center but sometimes in an outpatient clinic or during a religious or cultural ceremony at a later date. For more information on this procedure, see page 17.

Consider a Home Health Care Visit

Because many new families are sent home shortly after childbirth, many parents feel that their babies could benefit from additional health care during the first few days at home. Newborn jaundice, umbilical cord care, skin care, and feeding issues are common concerns. If you think you'd like some professional postpartum support, consider arranging a home health care visit soon after you arrive home from the hospital or birth center. Nurses with maternal-newborn training can help you care for your baby and advise you when further medical attention is needed. Some health care plans cover all or a portion of the expense; check to see whether yours does. Other helpful professionals include lactation consultants, who can help you learn to breastfeed, and postpartum doulas, specially trained laypeople who take care of you and your home so you can focus on your baby.

Establish a Support System

After you give birth, you'll discover a new world with your baby. The physical and emotional changes you'll experience, along with the increased responsibility, may leave you feeling overwhelmed. And the desire to do everything "right," from feeding and bathing your baby to keeping the toilets scrubbed, can only increase the pressure.

Don't feel you have to brave parenthood alone. Arranging for help and setting up a support system *before* your baby arrives will ensure that you can manage—and enjoy—the first few weeks with your little one. Think now about the kind of help you'll need. For example, you may want:

- Help with baby care, including breastfeeding, bathing, comforting, and so on
- Help with household tasks, like meal preparation and laundry
- Transportation to medical appointments, the grocery store or pharmacy, and so on
- Companionship

Ask for help whenever you need it; this isn't the time to be reserved. And always remember this advice: If someone trustworthy offers you help, whether it's to watch your baby so you can take a quick shower or to drive you to the grocery store, *take the offer*!

> If your baby arrives earlier than expected or has unanticipated issues, such as fever or jaundice, make sure you are clearly informed about the special care and support that will be necessary. See appendix for recommended resources.

Take Care of Practical Needs

Make sure you've borrowed, bought, or acquired as many of the items you will need before the birth, because taking a newborn on shopping trips or outings can be daunting! Throughout this book, you'll find information to help you make safe, sensible choices that will best prepare you for parenthood. On pages 29–31 you'll find tips to help you decide what type of diapers to use. On pages 51–55 are recommendations for dressing a new baby. On pages 117–21, you'll learn about what to look for when buying equipment for your child, including extra information on car seat and crib safety.

Chapter One

Your Newborn

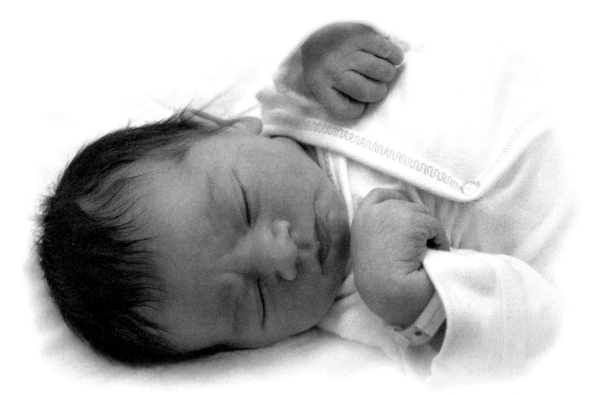

If you're a new parent, you probably spent lots of time learning about pregnancy and childbirth and worrying how you'd handle labor and delivery. You longed to hold your healthy baby in your arms. These memories of pregnancy and childbirth won't soon fade. (In fact, they'll grow and become more meaningful; you might find yourself telling any willing listener the detailed story of your child's birth!) But once your child is born, you realize childbirth was the beginning of parenthood, not just the end of pregnancy.

This year with your baby will be full of firsts—the first smile, the first tooth, the first word, and maybe even the first step. Your baby will need a lot of your care and attention as she accomplishes these and other firsts. A year from now, you'll be amazed by how much your child has grown and changed (likely more than any other year of her life), and you'll be proud of how much you've learned and accomplished as a parent. A new baby is famous for making life unpredictable. In the middle of a quiet dinner or long-overdue lovemaking or a much-needed phone conversation with a supportive friend, your baby suddenly needs you *now*. And you go to her—gladly. Few things in life are more satisfying than comforting and nurturing your child.

Here are some changes you and your family can expect when your newborn arrives.

Parents

Let's face it: Becoming a parent means you'll have less free time and fewer opportunities to be spontaneous. Going to a movie or a restaurant will almost never happen without a lot of preplanning. You'll need to arrange child care and work around your baby's schedule, not just your own. Plus, you'll wonder how long you can stay away from your little one. Once you walk out the door without your baby, you'll find yourself thinking and talking of nothing but her.

If you're parenting with a partner, a newborn can test a couple's relationship—especially if the baby is your first. To you both, it may seem as though the entire day—and night—consists of diapering and feeding and rocking and burping. You may feel as though you're losing touch with each other. Your partner may even feel a bit jealous of the attention you're giving the baby. Know that it takes time to adjust to parenthood. Once you've grown used to your roles as parents, find ways and time to nurture your relationship. Remember: You're in this together!

If you're parenting without a partner, you might feel overwhelmed at first. You may be exhausted, and not having anyone to share the work, frustrations, and joys with may make your new role seem that much more difficult. Be sure to establish a support system. Having family and friends to look after your baby occasionally, or just listen to you, will help greatly. You might also consider joining a single-mothers group. See the appendix to learn more about single-mother support networks.

Mom

Both parents experience emotional ups and downs during the first weeks of their baby's life, but moms are especially vulnerable during the postpartum days. Lack of sleep, tremendous hormonal changes, and feelings of being overwhelmed can cause bouts of depression.

For some, these emotional fluctuations are mild and subside within a few weeks ("baby blues"). Eating right, gradually exercising more often, and sleeping when the baby sleeps usually help chase away baby blues. Supportive family, friends, and other new parents can help new moms feel back on track.

For others, however, the emotional fluctuations are overwhelming, long lasting, and may require treatment. These women may suffer from postpartum mood disorders (PPMDs) or postpartum psychosis. Make sure you talk with your health care provider if your depression concerns you or those around you. He or she will have ways to help you.

Dad or Other Parent

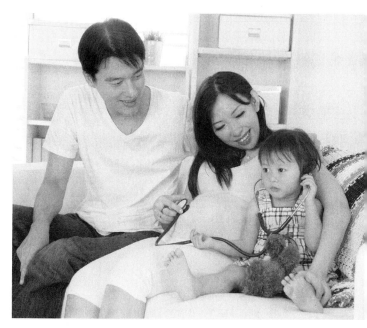

Although a new dad or other parent doesn't experience the hormonal and physical changes that a new mom does, he or she may experience a range of emotions. Confusion, ambivalence, fear, depression—these are all emotions they can feel about their new role, even while feeling an intense love for the baby.

Just as with new moms, supportive family, friends, and other new parents can help these parents.

Siblings

If you have an older child, no matter how well you've prepared her for the baby's arrival, she may still have trouble accepting the fact that she's no longer the baby. She may suddenly want to start nursing again. Her sleep patterns may change. She may start sucking her thumb or wetting herself. These regressions are normal and simply her way of seeking the love and attention she fears the baby will steal from her. To help reassure her, spend (and see that your partner spends) some uninterrupted one-on-one time with your older child every day. Listen carefully to her feelings about the baby and the changes in your family. Point out the benefits of being an older child, like choosing what to eat, being able to go to the park to play, and having friends.

Today, many babies are born into families that don't fit the once traditional mold—that is, a working dad and a stay-at-home mom who are married to each other. Lots of moms return to work after their maternity leave, and more and more dads are choosing to care for their babies full time at home. Many single men and women want to know the joys of parenting and choose to adopt a child. Some single women might opt to become pregnant on their own, and a single man might work with a surrogate. An increasing number of same-sex couples are becoming loving parents, and the number of blended families is also on the rise. Furthermore, not every baby born to a family is without problems. A baby may be born prematurely or have some kind of medical problem, like alcohol or street drugs in her system. She may be born with a genetic condition or a congenital problem, like Down's syndrome or a cleft palate. Whatever the family's structure and however a baby joins the family, every parent should pledge to provide a loving, safe, and healthy environment for the little one as she enters our increasingly global community. (For further helpful information, see the recommended resources in the appendix.)

Changes for the Baby

While parents must adjust to life with their newborn, a baby must adjust to life outside her mom's womb. Being born, whether vaginally or by cesarean section, is an exhausting physical experience. In fact, after an initial alert period at birth, most newborns fall into a deep sleep for about six hours.

Here are other changes a baby undergoes after birth:

- At birth, a baby normally weighs between six and eight pounds (2.7 and 3.6 kilograms) and is eighteen to twenty-two inches (45.7 to 55.9 centimeters) long. Typically, she'll lose up to 10 percent of her weight in the days following birth, then start to regain that weight by the end of the first week.

- While in the womb, a baby receives all her nourishment through the umbilical cord. She doesn't have to swallow to satisfy her hunger. In fact, she doesn't know what hunger is! Once born, swallowing becomes a reflex, and the baby feels hunger and knows she must act to satisfy it.

- Before birth, a baby doesn't breathe. She receives all her oxygen through her mom's blood. At birth, her circulation is sluggish, and her breathing may be shallow and irregular (although her heart may beat 120 times per minute). She'll also sneeze, gasp, hiccup, and cough. These aren't cold symptoms; they're just her way of clearing mucus from the respiratory system.

- In the womb, amniotic fluid keeps a baby at a constant comfortable temperature. Once born, however, her temperature drops rapidly. To warm her, health care providers will place her on her mom's chest or abdomen and covered with a blanket or swaddled. (Alternatively, she may be placed in or under a warmer.)

- In the womb, the surrounding fluid, blood, and tissue muffled outside sounds and kept the baby "in the dark." Once born, however, she experiences sounds much more loudly and clearly, and she's exposed to direct, bright light. Before birth, her sleeping and waking schedules were her own and weren't influenced by the light of day and dark of night.

- Before birth, a baby was constantly and gently rocked by her mother's movements, a motion she found calming and reassuring. After birth, she must rely on others to remember to provide this motion. (This is why rocking a fussy baby can calm her.)

With all these changes, it's little wonder that babies spend much of their first few weeks sleeping and adjusting to their new surroundings and their new abilities.

What Does a Newborn Look Like?

Contrary to popular belief, not all newborns are cute. In fact, many can look downright peculiar. Following are descriptions of a typical newborn's features in the days immediately following birth.

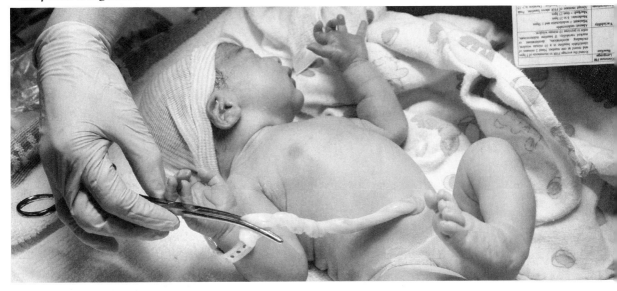

Head, Hair, and Neck

A newborn's head is large in proportion to her body—about one-fourth of her body's length—making her quite "top heavy" with little or no head control. Her neck is short and creased. Her head may look lopsided, and the top of it may appear pointy (this "molding" is caused by the skull bones shifting to allow for a smoother passage through the birth canal). The head usually regains a rounded shape a couple of days after birth. A tough membrane protects the head's two soft spots, called fontanels, where the skull bones haven't yet fused (allowing brain growth to continue). Your care provider will monitor brain growth and ventricle (fluid chambers within the brain) size by measuring your baby's head circumference in addition to height and weight. The anterior fontanel, the larger one at the top near the front, closes after eighteen to twenty-four months. It is not abnormal to be able to see pulsing at the site of the anterior fontanel. The posterior fontanel, at the top near the back, closes by six months.

It's impossible to predict how much hair newborns will have or keep. Some have lots of locks and may never lose them. Others have no hair or a short crop that will fall out and regrow after about six weeks, sometimes in a completely different color. Some newborns have wrinkly scalps and will eventually grow into the extra skin. Others may have peeling scalps (cradle cap).

Face

A newborn's eyes often appear red and puffy, and there may be broken blood vessels in her eyeballs. This is caused by pressure exerted on them during birth or by the drops or ointment she received after birth to prevent infection. Light-skinned babies usually have blue-gray eyes, and dark-skinned babies usually have brown eyes. Permanent color might not develop for about six months. Some babies can produce tears from birth, but most don't for six weeks or so.

A newborn's nose appears flat and broad. For the first five months or so, she is an "obligate" nose breather, meaning she needs to breathe primarily through her nose.

Occasionally babies are born with teeth, called natal teeth. They can cause pain and interfere with breastfeeding; your baby's care provider or dentist may need to remove them. Blisters may be present on the lips from in utero sucking; these are normal and aren't painful. Babies are often born with a white spot on the center of the roof of the mouth, called an Epstein pearl. This is normal and will resolve spontaneously over the next few weeks.

A newborn usually has fat cheeks, and she may appear chinless.

Skin/Fingernails

A newborn's skin is wrinkled and loose, and it may begin to look dry and start to peel after a few days. Her body may be covered with vernix caseosa, a white, waxy substance that eased her movement through the birth canal. She may also still have lanugo, a downy fuzz covering her shoulders, back, and cheeks. This soft hair will disappear within a few days.

Skin color usually changes during the first few days, ranging from bluish purple to pink to gray. Newborns of African, Asian, or Mediterranean descent often have light skin that will darken eventually. A blue color of the lips, gums, or skin around the mouth may represent a deficiency of oxygen in these tissues and should be evaluated.

Fingernails can be long and sharp, and grow fast, and are likely to result in scratches on the face as the newborn has little control over stray movements. (See page 42 for how to trim your baby's nails.)

Body

A newborn's body curls into itself, and her abdomen is large and her hips narrow. After birth, a metal or plastic clamp is placed low on her umbilical cord before the cord is cut. The clamp stops the bleeding from the umbilical vessels and is removed before she leaves the hospital or birth center. The remaining stump of tissue will fall off on its own. Your baby's care provider or the staff at the hospital or birth center will tell you how to care for the stump. (See page 40 to learn more.) Whether your baby ends up with an "innie" or "outie" belly button is out of your control; it depends on how the cord heals.

Whether a girl or a boy, a newborn's breasts and genitalia may be swollen, and the nipples may even leak a milky substance, sometimes referred to as "witch's milk." Baby girls may slightly bleed or discharge mucus from the vagina. The presence of maternal hormones in the newborn causes these effects, which most often disappear in a few days or weeks.

Some babies are born with extra nipples (called supernumerary or accessory nipples) or extra breast tissue located on the chest or abdomen below the regular nipple line. These are no cause for medical concern. Cosmetic concerns can be addressed much later.

Arms

A newborn's arms are flexed. The hands, which are generally cool and curled into fists, may look blue because of an immature circulatory system. The wrists may be fat and creased.

Legs

A newborn's knees are bent, and the legs are bowed. A newborn's immature circulatory system may make the feet, like the hands, look blue. A newborn's feet are also mottled and may appear flat because of fat pads on the soles.

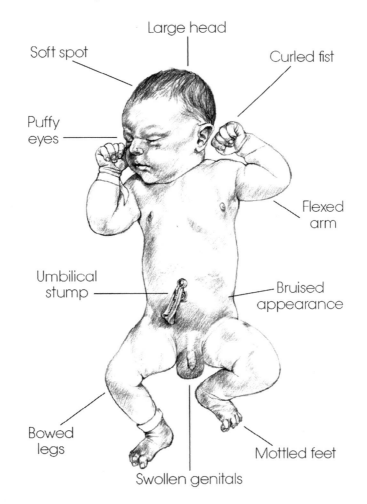

Large head

Soft spot

Curled fist

Puffy eyes

Flexed arm

Umbilical stump

Bruised appearance

Bowed legs

Mottled feet

Swollen genitals

Conditions That May Be Present at Birth

Even after an uncomplicated birth, your baby may have one or more of the following conditions. These conditions may be present at birth, and they most often heal or disappear with time.

Types of Birthmarks

Some birthmarks may be present at birth, while others may develop in the first month. They're very common, and most of them shouldn't cause concern. Most birthmarks disappear or fade on their own by the time a child is five or six.

Nevi (moles)

These are usually small, dark-brown to black spots that can be present at birth or appear later. They can be flat or raised. Very rarely, a baby's born with a large nevus, which a dermatologist should check. Nevi can grow as the child grows, and while they rarely become cancerous later, it's a good idea to monitor their appearance for life.

Café-au-Lait Spots

Light-brown marks known as "café au lait" (coffee with cream) spots also may be present. These usually require no intervention but may need further evaluation if they're unusually large or more than six are present.

Hemangiomas (blood vessel malformations)

- Flat angiomata ("salmon patches"): These may also be referred to as nevus flammeus. Often called "angel kisses" (if they appear between the eyes) or "stork bites" (if they're at the back of the neck), these flat pink or light-red patches are the most common birthmarks. They're usually on or around the eyelids, forehead, bridge of the nose, or on the back of the head and neck. They may darken with crying or straining, but they usually fade in a few months.

- Capillary hemangiomas ("strawberry" marks): These bumps aren't usually noticeable at birth but appear in the first month as small raised dots. They grow fairly rapidly during the first six months and then begin to shrink, eventually disappearing most often by age five or six.

- Port-wine stains: These are irregularly shaped dark-red or purple spots that sometimes fade but don't disappear completely. If they're around the eye or forehead, they may need further evaluation because of potential associated health problems.

- Mongolian spots: These flat black, gray, brown, or bluish areas are common on darker-skinned newborns, most frequently on the back or buttocks. These spots can be large or small, and most disappear by age five or six. These spots can look like bruises, but they're not caused by trauma.

Milia/Miliaria

Milia are undeveloped or blocked sweat glands that usually look like white or yellow pinpoint spots on the nose, chin, and cheeks. They disappear over time, usually over the first weeks of life.

Miliaria (also known as prickly heat) is another name for heat rash, which can show up as fine pink pimples usually on the face or in skin folds. If your baby is affected, give her frequent cool baths or sponge baths to help open her pores. Sweating from overwrapping may cause miliaria, so the best prevention is to keep your baby dry and at a comfortable temperature.

Newborn Rashes

Within a few days after birth, many newborns develop a very common rash called erythema toxicum. This appears as a red splotch with a yellowish-white center. These splotches or pimples often appear on the chest, back, or face and usually disappear within a few days without treatment.

Another benign newborn rash is neonatal pustular melanosis. It produces small blisters that dry and peel, leaving freckle-like marks. It is most common in babies with darker skin. Sometimes a blistering rash can also indicate an infection, so it is best to have blisters checked.

In general, it is normal for the skin to become dry and then crack and peel within the first week. This will resolve by itself.

Newborn Jaundice

Jaundice is a common condition in newborns. It's caused by the liver's inability to efficiently process the by-products of old, broken-down red blood cells (bilirubin), giving the skin and the whites of the eyes a yellowish color. Newborns are born with lots of red blood cells and often immature livers that are slow to process large amounts of bilirubin. (After processing through the liver, bilirubin is eliminated in the stool.) This condition often appears within a few days after birth and disappears once the liver becomes more efficient (usually a week after birth).

If jaundice appears within the first twenty-four hours after birth, it might be related to a difference in blood types between you and your baby and may need closer monitoring and more aggressive treatment. Regardless, your baby will be observed closely in the hospital or birth center for the development of jaundice. It usually presents in a head-to-toe direction. Typically, the lower on the body the jaundice appears, the higher the level of bilirubin.

Because jaundice often appears after babies leave the hospital or birth center, your baby's care provider should check her a few days after birth to look for signs of jaundice. Sometimes a care provider will monitor a newborn's bilirubin level with blood tests. In many cases, no treatment is necessary. Parents need only to make sure their child is feeding well and peeing and pooping often, and to watch for any signs that the condition is worsening (for example, the skin and eyes stay or become more yellow, the baby develops a high-pitched cry, or she becomes sluggish and irritable). If the jaundice persists or worsens, the newborn may receive phototherapy (light treatment). The blue lights used in phototherapy have a particular wavelength that has been shown to speed up bilirubin breakdown. Your baby might be placed directly under these blue lights or covered with a biliblanket, a portable phototherapy device that bathes the baby in light. Although rare, severe jaundice, if left untreated, can cause hearing loss, mental retardation, and behavior problems.

Although breastfed babies may acquire jaundice more often than formula-fed babies, *this is usually not a reason to discontinue breastfeeding.* Sometimes the condition results when the baby doesn't consume enough breast milk and becomes dehydrated, either because she's having trouble latching on or because the milk supply is low. In either case, more frequent feedings and getting help with breastfeeding should increase the baby's milk consumption. Other times, the condition results when breast milk affects the elimination of bilirubin (breast-milk jaundice). Usually, the jaundice gradually decreases, but breastfed babies can have mild jaundice for several weeks. This condition is rarely harmful, and most often care providers recommend that moms continue to breastfeed exclusively, although it's possible a care provider may recommend that a mom interrupt breastfeeding for a day or two to let her baby's bilirubin levels decrease. In this case, she should pump her breasts to maintain a steady milk supply. (See pages 78–79.)

Lip Blisters
Your baby's intense sucking may cause a blister on her lips. These are normal and not painful.

Tears and Blocked Tear Ducts
The lacrimal system that makes and drains tears (which serve an important function in protecting the eye's surface) is not fully developed at birth, and it may be months before your baby cries "real tears." Some babies are born with a condition called dacryostenosis, in which the tear ducts are blocked and don't drain effectively, leading to excessive tearing or even discharge in the affected eye(s). Usually the ducts open on their own. Sometimes massaging the ducts (ask your care provider how to do this) or cleaning them with moist compresses will help clear the discharge. If the blocked ducts persist, a minor surgical procedure may be needed near the end of the first year to open the ducts.

Broken Collarbone (Clavicle)
A vaginal birth sometimes breaks a baby's clavicle. It'll heal in a few weeks, even without special treatment. A small lump will probably appear at the fracture site, but it'll later disappear on its own. Being aware of the break when lifting a newborn will prevent her discomfort.

Dislocated Hips (Developmental Dysplasia of the Hips)
Babies may be born with or develop abnormalities involving instability or looseness of the hip joint. Babies, especially girls, who have been in a breech or bottom-first position are at a higher risk. The condition may be detected on the first exam or in the days and weeks following birth. You should notify your baby's care provider if you have a family history

of early childhood hip problems. During your baby's first year, her care provider will examine her for this condition during routine well-child checkups and treat it if necessary.

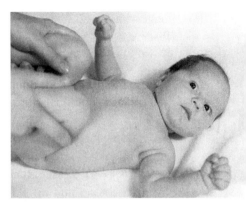

Swellings of the Head (Cephalohematoma/Caput Succedaneum)

A cephalohematoma or a caput succedaneum is a swelling of blood beneath the scalp. Bruising may be present as well. It occurs when a baby's head presses against the pelvic bone during a vaginal birth, or when a baby is delivered by vacuum extraction or forceps. Your newborn may have one or several big "goose eggs" at the top or back of the scalp, and some may become hard. These may increase bilirubin production and can be a contributing factor for jaundice, but shouldn't cause other problems. They usually disappear in about a week.

Buttocks Crease Dimple (Sacral Dimple)

It's not uncommon for a baby to have a dimple located at the top of or just below her buttocks crease. Usually this is shallow and of no consequence, but it may be an indicator of underlying developmental problems of the spine or spinal cord. Your care provider will let you know if any further evaluation is indicated.

Bulging of Skin in Groin Area (Inguinal Hernia)

A groin or inguinal hernia develops when a small opening in the lining or wall of the abdomen allows part of the intestine to bulge outward—in boys into the scrotum (testicular sac) and in girls into the groin. It is much more common in premature babies and in boys. The groin or scrotum will appear larger than usual on one or both sides and will likely enlarge even further when the baby is crying (due to pressure from within). Surgery is usually done to prevent the intestine from becoming stuck, swollen, or twisted outside the abdomen.

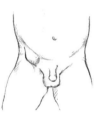

Bulge in Skin around the Belly Button (Umbilical Hernia)

Some babies will have a persistent opening in the abdominal wall muscle, called an umbilical hernia, near the navel. Tissue from within the abdomen may bulge outward, especially when the baby cries. Most of the time, this opening gradually closes on its own. There is no need to try to keep the tissue from coming in and out.

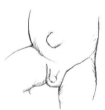

Swollen Testicles (Hydrocele)

A hydrocele is a swelling from excess fluid around a baby boy's testicle(s). It can mimic a hernia because the testicle appears large. To uncover whether your baby has a hydrocele or a hernia, your care provider may hold a light next to the scrotum. If it glows, it will suggest the swelling is from fluid, not the intestine. Your care provider may continue to observe it, but hydroceles usually disappear without treatment within the first year.

Abnormal Location of Urinary Opening (Hypospadias)

Some baby boys are born with the penile opening for urine (the urethra or meatus) located on the underside, rather than at the tip, of the penis. This often requires corrective surgery at a later time (most commonly done around twelve to eighteen months of age). These babies should not be circumcised because the foreskin tissue may be needed for the procedure.

Absence of Testicles within the Scrotum (Undescended Testes)

Normally, a baby boy's testes descend into the scrotum in utero, and their presence can be felt at birth. Sometimes, however, one or both of the testicles is slow to descend and is located higher in the groin or even in the abdomen at the time of birth. If the testicles do not proceed to descend on their own, surgery may be indicated later in the first or second year.

Misshapen Feet/Curved Legs

Having feet that appear turned, misshapen, or "pigeon toed" is common in newborns because of their position in the uterus. This condition (also called intoeing) usually corrects itself before the end of the first year. Most care providers don't recommend treatment in the first year unless there are also other foot deformities. If the feet are rigid or can't be straightened with movement, or if there are underlying bone abnormalities, casting or surgery may be necessary.

Tongue-Tie (Ankyloglossia)

With this condition, the cord of tissue (frenulum) attaching a newborn's tongue to the floor of her mouth may be shorter and tauter than usual, limiting the tongue's forward movement. In rare cases, cutting the frenulum may be suggested to correct the problem if it interferes with effective latch on.

Wrist Sores (Lesions)

Newborns can produce lesions by sucking on their wrists while in the womb. They'll disappear without treatment over time.

Newborn Exams and Procedures

Your newborn will be examined in the hospital or birth center for a variety of reasons. Some exams and procedures take place immediately after birth in the delivery room, and some are delayed until just before you head home, when your baby is more settled. These routine procedures are no cause for alarm, and which ones are required may vary from state to state. Contact your state's Department of Health to learn which tests it requires. If you have any questions about these tests, discuss them with your care provider ahead of time.

Drying Off and Skin-to-Skin Contact

If you have a vaginal birth, your baby will be dried off immediately after the birth and should be placed on your stomach. This skin-to-skin contact will help warm your baby and start the bonding process. If you plan on breastfeeding, this is a good time to begin. In many hospitals, evaluations can take place while you hold your baby.

If you have a cesarean birth, your baby will likely be dried off by a member of the medical staff while you're getting stitched up. Once the staff suctions her mouth and nose, and performs the necessary evaluations, your baby can be placed on your stomach for skin-to-skin contact. If you're too tired, your partner may be able to hold your baby to his or her skin. You can begin to bond with your baby and breastfeed once you've recovered.

Cord Clamping

After delivery, the umbilical cord will still be attached to the placenta. It may pulsate as it continues to provide oxygen to your baby as she begins to take her first breaths. Within a short period of time, the cord will be clamped and cut. The clamp will be removed in the next day or two, after it has dried. The remaining stump will fall off in the next weeks.

Cord Blood Banking

Cord blood contains primitive early blood cells (stem cells) that can be sent in a preordered kit to a cord blood bank for private use, for public use (donation), or for research. If you have a close family member or relative with a disease that may require a bone marrow transplant as treatment, it might be helpful to arrange to

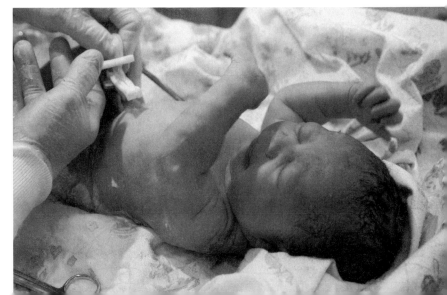

store blood in a private bank. Otherwise, the American Academy of Pediatrics (AAP) does not recommend collecting and storing cord blood in private banks at this time. You may want to consider donating the stem cells for public use and research. This is free and easy to do.

Eye Care

When a baby passes through the birth canal, her eyes may catch any infections the mother is carrying there. Some infections can cause blindness, so to prevent them a care provider commonly administers eye drops or erythromycin ointment in the newborn's eyes.

Vitamin K Shot

Shortly after birth, a care provider will inject your baby with vitamin K, which increases her body's ability to clot blood. This shot is meant to prevent serious bleeding problems until your baby can process vitamin K on her own.

Apgar Tests

Immediately after the birth, a care provider will evaluate your baby using the Apgar scale (see below), which indicates your baby's well-being and responsiveness. The care provider will observe your baby's heart rate, respiratory effort, muscle tone, reflex irritability (or response), and skin color. Then he or she will record a score of zero to two for each of these five areas, first at one minute and again at five minutes after birth. Don't be overly concerned about your baby's performance: A perfect score of ten is unusual, and scores over seven are just fine. Even lower scores are seldom cause for alarm.

Sign	0	1	2
Heart Rate	Absent	Slow (Under 100 beats per minute)	Normal (Over 100 beats per minute)
Respiratory Effort	Absent	Slow, irregular	Good, crying
Muscle Tone	Limp, floppy	Some flexing of extremities	Active, spontaneous motion
Reflex Irritability (Response to catheter or bulb syringe in nostril)	No response	Grimace	Cough or sneeze
Color	Blue, pale	Body pink, extremities blue	Completely pink

Identification

Soon after delivery, a nurse will put a bracelet or tag on you and your baby for identification purposes. She or he also may take a footprint of your baby.

Newborn Exam

Typically, a care provider will examine your baby thoroughly within twenty-four hours of birth. If you're in the hospital more than one day, your baby will likely get a full discharge examination before heading home. Exams provide an excellent opportunity for you to ask questions and learn. The care provider will check your baby from head to toe for birth-marks, check her eyes to make sure there are no cataracts, listen to her heartbeat, feel her pulses, test for developmental problems of the hips, check her reflexes (see pages 21–22), and examine the inner organs that can be felt through her soft skin. The care provider may also conclude whether your baby is preterm or post-term by determining more exactly what her gestational age is.

Hepatitis B Vaccination

Hepatitis B is a serious disease that attacks the liver and can lead to cirrhosis or liver cancer. Since vaccination started in 1991, rates of infection in children have dropped by more than 95 percent. Vaccination guidelines state that babies should receive the first dose of the vaccine at birth, the second dose between ages one and two months, and the third dose between ages six and eighteen months. Babies whose mothers have tested positive for hepatitis B should be given an additional shot (hepatitis B immune globulin). Consult with your baby's care provider.

Screening Blood Tests

A care provider will check your baby for several diseases that could cause serious damage but don't have any visible symptoms so might be otherwise missed. He or she will obtain a blood sample by pricking your baby's heel sometime after twenty-four hours of age and send it to a state public health laboratory for analysis. Which specific tests and how many are screened for varies from state to state. Check with your state's Department of Health or the National Newborn Screening and Genetics Regulation Center (NNSGRC) website: http://www.genes-r-us.uthscsa.edu/. The March of Dimes also has information and a video about the importance of newborn screening on their website (http://www.marchofdimes .com). The Centers for Disease Control and Prevention (CDC) provides information on any of these diseases as well: http://www.cdc.gov/newbornscreening.

Following are the most common diseases for which newborns are screened:

- Phenylketonuria (PKU): Affecting one infant in twelve thousand, PKU is a hereditary disease that's caused by the body's inability to digest protein normally. Unaffected parents can pass on PKU, which causes mental retardation and organ damage if not treated. Newborns with this disease shouldn't be breastfed (although consuming a very small amount of breast milk may be okay with a care provider's approval). Instead, they're put on a special formula that's low in phenylalanine, the part of the protein that the body can't digest.

- Galactosemia: This hereditary disease occurs when the body can't use milk sugar (lactose). Unaffected parents can pass on the disease, which affects one infant in fifty thousand. Newborns with this disease can't be breastfed and must drink a lactose-free formula. If babies are not diagnosed early enough, galactosemia can cause mental retardation, cataracts, and an enlarged liver.

- Hypothyroidism: A defect in the thyroid gland causes hypothyroidism, which is treatable with hormone medication. This condition affects one infant in four thousand and, if left untreated, causes growth problems, mental retardation, and lethargy.
- Congenital adrenal hyperplasia: This disease is a genetic disorder that results in a hormonal imbalance and affects one infant in fifteen thousand. It can cause sexual development problems, hormone problems, and death if not treated with replacement hormones.
- Hemoglobinopathy: This disease causes changes in red blood cells. Sickle-cell disease is the most common form of hemoglobinopathy, and it can cause anemia (a low red blood cell count) as well as other serious problems. Sickle-cell disease usually affects those of African, Mediterranean, Indian, or Middle Eastern descent, but anyone is susceptible. This test can also detect other forms of hemoglobinopathy. Some forms of the disease require medical monitoring and intervention, while others require no treatment.
- Other metabolic disorders: Screening tests can also detect other diseases, including cystic fibrosis and many metabolic conditions like maple syrup urine disease, biotinidase deficiency, and fatty acid oxidation disorders.

Newborn Hearing Screening

The American Academy of Pediatrics (AAP) recommends that all newborns get tested for hearing loss before leaving the hospital or birth center. Severe to profound hearing loss affects one to six newborns out of one thousand, and many affected babies don't have any risk factors that would prompt screening. Intervention for hearing loss is available and recommended by six months of age. A care provider will use one of the two following procedures to test your baby's hearing:

- Auditory brainstem response (ABR) test: This test measures how the brain responds to sounds.
- Otoacoustic emissions (OAE) test: This test measures sound waves produced in the inner ear.

Both procedures are quick (about five to ten minutes), painless, noninvasive, and can be done while your baby is sleeping or lying still. If you don't receive the results before heading home, call your care provider's office to confirm them. If you can't have your newborn's hearing screened at the hospital, you should have it done before she is three months old. See page 188 for possible warning signs of hearing loss.

Newborn Critical Congenital Heart Disease Screening

Approximately one hundred to two hundred children die each year of complications of various types of critical congenital heart disease. In an effort to improve early recognition of these conditions, the AAP (American Academy of Pediatrics) and other organizations are recommending that all newborns are screened. This is done with a test called pulse oximetry; it is painless and noninvasive. A sensor is placed on a thin part of the body (like an infant's toes). The sensor then measures the oxygen delivery to that area. Further testing will be done if the results are not normal.

Circumcision

Circumcision is a surgical procedure that removes some of the skin that covers the tip of the penis (foreskin). This procedure should be performed by an experienced person (medical professional or religious officiant), and it usually happens before the baby leaves the hospital or birth center but sometimes in an outpatient clinic or during a religious or cultural ceremony at a later date.

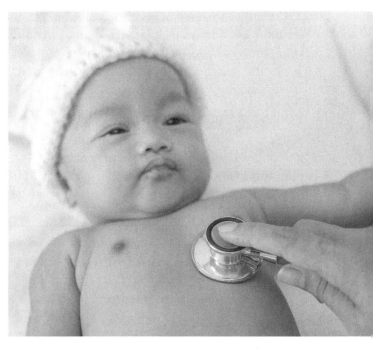

This procedure is not required by any health care organization in the United States. The American Academy of Pediatrics has weighed in with the following statement: "Circumcision has potential medical benefits and advantages, as well as risks. Evaluation of current evidence indicates that the health benefits of newborn male circumcision outweigh the risks and that the procedure's benefits justify access to this procedure for families who choose it, however, existing scientific evidence is not sufficient to recommend routine circumcision. Therefore, because the procedure is not essential to a child's current well-being, we recommend that the decision to circumcise is one best made by parents in consultation with their pediatrician, taking into account what is in the best interests of the child, including medical, religious, cultural, and ethnic traditions." Ask your care provider about the pros and cons of circumcision before your baby's birth. Research the topic on your own. If circumcision is part of your culture or religious tradition, talk to a respected leader about the meaning behind it and reasons for the procedure. Consider as much information as you can before making your decision.

The pros for circumcision include potential medical benefits: lowering the risk of urinary tract infections (UTIs), penile cancer, human immunodeficiency virus (HIV), and human papillomavirus (HPV). Other reasons for circumcision stem from religious traditions (such as the Jewish bris), social customs, and cultural beliefs.

Those who oppose circumcision believe that its risks outweigh its potential benefits. The risks include pain, infection, bleeding, and mutilation.

If you decide to have your baby circumcised, the AAP recommends that he be given an analgesic before the procedure to block pain. A premature or ill baby, or one with an abnormally developed penis, should not be circumcised. Bleeding problems and infection are more likely to occur. Also, make sure you notify your care provider ahead of time if your family has a history of bleeding problems.

In the United States, it is currently estimated that 55 percent of newborn boys are circumcised.

Leaving the Hospital

Every newborn should meet certain criteria before he or she is deemed okay to be discharged from the hospital or birth-place setting. The following table provides a list of these guidelines. Also, it is very important that arrangements are made for follow-up within forty-eight hours of discharge either with a home health care visit or a clinic appointment.

Newborn Hospital Discharge Recommendations from the AAP

1. A normal clinical and physical exam is done.
2. Two successful feedings have been completed by the newborn.
3. An appropriate car seat is available and training on correct use has taken place.
4. Risk factors have been reviewed for the family, environment, and social situation.
5. You've chosen a pediatrician or care provider for ongoing care.

Your Newborn's World

Until recently, researchers thought newborns were naturally passive and uninterested in their environment. Today, they're learning that newborns are remarkably responsive and perceive the world almost as well as adults—and in some cases, better than adults. Here are brief descriptions of a newborn's senses and faculties.

Touch

Before birth, touch lets a baby relate to her surroundings more than any other sense. Once born, a newborn is still very sensitive to touch, probably more so than adults. She can perceive small changes in texture or temperature, and she loves warm, soft, firm pressure, especially on the front of her body. Being swaddled (see pages 25–26) or held closely often calms her, and your baby may find a light, gentle massage extremely soothing and comforting (see page 41). Make sure you always place your baby on her back when she is swaddled, and monitor her so she does not roll over. Swaddling should be discontinued before the baby is trying to roll herself over, usually around two months.

Close physical contact between parent and baby in the first weeks can promote a newborn's sense of well-being and aids her development in ways that can be measured several years afterward. Breastfeeding lets a mother begin to bond with her child within minutes or hours of birth. Cuddling, kissing, stroking, lots of eye-to-eye and skin-to-skin contact, and other affectionate interactions are wonderful ways for both parents to begin their relationship with their newborn. Because contact is so important, many hospitals and birth centers have relaxed routine procedures so they don't interfere with this bonding. Before you choose your birth place, ask your care provider whether rooming-in will be possible.

Sight

Although newborns can see at birth, they best see objects that are about six to ten inches away. This is the distance between a baby's face and her parent's face during feeding or cuddling. Beyond that distance, newborns see only brightness and movement, and many have crossed eyes, which is a normal condition in early infancy (see page 169).

Newborn eyes may track an object moving slowly from side to side or, with more difficulty, an object moving up and down. By the time your baby is two months old, her eyes should track objects that move slowly in any direction. If you have any concerns about your baby's sight, ask her care provider to test her vision.

Newborns observe the world with unlimited interest. They'll often stop feeding to stare at objects, especially patterned objects and those with sharply contrasting colors. Soon they'll rather look at faces than anything else.

Hearing

Most babies are born with well-developed hearing. Within ten minutes after birth, a baby can locate a sound source, and she seems to prefer high-pitched voices and rhythmic, soft sounds. Loud noises should startle a newborn or make her move (see page 21). She seems to respond to sounds that last at least ten seconds. Sometimes, a sound will intrigue her so much that she'll stop feeding to pay more attention to it. If you have any concerns about how your baby responds to sounds, ask her care provider to test her hearing.

Smell and Taste

Researchers know little about a newborn's sense of smell or taste, mostly because it's difficult to tell when a baby discriminates between one smell or taste and another. Foul odors usually upset a newborn. And she seems to react to sweet, sour, and salty tastes and can differentiate among plain, slightly sweetened, and very sweet water.

Intelligence

Babies are born with a keen, discriminating interest in their environment. They can choose to pay attention to one object and ignore others. They soon can combine touch, sight, and hearing into meaningful patterns.

At first, a newborn's short memory won't let her remember an object if it doesn't reappear within two and a half seconds. She reacts with her whole body to various stimuli and changes in her environment, like a drop in temperature or a loud noise.

Sociability

Although babies are only aware of their own existence, they find people interesting. They crave eye, vocal, and physical contact with others, especially their parents. By the end of the first week, a newborn might recognize a parent's voice, and by two weeks she may know her parents by sight. By the end of the first month, she may behave differently with her parents than with other people. Some newborn babies smile either during sleep or when awake, though it's likely not intentional.

Reflexes during the First Year

A newborn's reflexes are spontaneous, automatic responses to external or internal stimuli. They're the building blocks of intelligence and the foundation of physical coordination. Some reflexes, like gagging and blinking, are lifelong. Others, like grasping and stepping, disappear or "go underground" only to reappear later as consciously controlled activities. Your baby's care provider will check for these reflexes to make sure she has a healthy nervous system.

Reflex	What Triggers It	Description	Appearance/ Disappearance
Startle (Moro)	External stimuli, like sudden changes in light, noise, movement, or position; Internal stimuli, like crying or muscle twitches during sleep.	A newborn will fling out the arms and legs, then quickly pull them into the chest while the body curls, as if to cling.	Tapers off in 1–2 mos. and disappears by 2–6 mos.
Sucking	Touching the roof of the baby's mouth or cheek with a nipple or finger	The baby's lips pucker while her tongue curls inward.	Is present before birth and strongest in the first 2 mos. After this it fades, merging gradually with voluntary activity.
Rooting (Searching)	Stroking a cheek or an area around the mouth	The baby's head turns in the direction of the stroking and searches with the lips for a nipple. The baby uses this reflex to seek food.	Continues while the baby is nursing, but usually gone by 4 mos.
Tongue Thrust (Extrusion)	Touching the baby's lips	The baby's tongue automatically moves forward when her lips are touched. This protects her from choking and aids feeding from the breast or bottle.	Often fades around 4 mos.
Grasping (Palmar, Plantar)	Stroking the palms of the hands or pressing the balls of the feet (at the bases of the toes)	The baby's fingers or toes curl as if to hold on to an object.	Decreases noticeably after 10 days and usually disappears around 5–6 mos. May continue in the feet until 9–12 mos.
Stepping	Holding the baby under the arms in a standing position and pressing down a little	The baby lifts each foot in turn, as if to walk.	Diminishes after 1 wk. and will disappear in about 2 mos. Recurs as voluntary walking around 1 yr.
Placing	Holding the baby's shins against an edge	The baby tries to step upward to put her feet on the surface of a table or bed.	Disappears in about 2 mos.

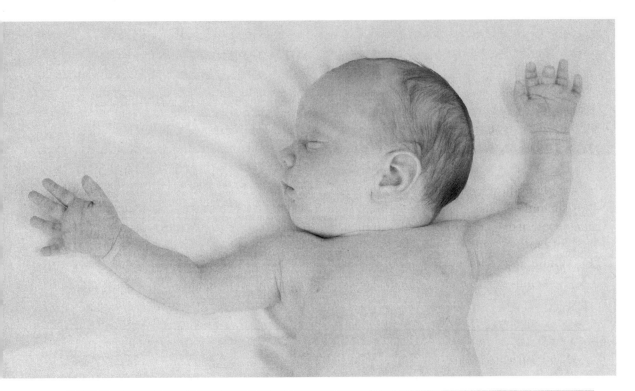

Reflex	What Triggers It	Description	Appearance/Disappearance
Tonic Neck (Fencing)	Laying the baby on her back	The baby's head is turned to one side while lying on her back. The arm on the side that the face is turned toward extends straight out, and the other arm flexes in a kind of fencer's pose.	Most obvious at 2–3 mos. and disappears at around 5–7 mos.
Blinking	Bright light, touching an eyelid, or sudden noise	The baby's eyelids open and close rapidly.	Permanent
Gagging	Foreign matter in the respiratory system	The baby chokes, gasps, spits up, and may turn blue. (Even when the head is under water, the reflex in most cases prevents infants from breathing in.)	Permanent
Swallowing	Food in the mouth	The baby's trachea closes while the esophagus opens.	Permanent
Withdrawal	Pain, cold air	The baby tries to pull away while drawing in her limbs close to the body.	Permanent
Parachute	"Diving" the baby toward the floor	The baby extends hands out for protection.	Appears around 7 mos. after birth

Chapter Two

Caring for Your Baby

Here are a few activities that are part of daily life with a newborn: feeding him, changing his diapers, dressing and undressing him, comforting him when he's fussy, and putting him to sleep. This routine won't change much during the first year. On his first birthday, your child will be just as incapable of changing his own diaper as he was when he was a week old.

When you change that first diaper, you may feel as helpless as your baby. You're nervous (especially if someone besides the baby is watching you), and each movement seems awkward and unnatural. Bath time may also give you the shakes, and dressing your baby for his first outing may seem to require at least four hands.

This chapter will help you handle these everyday tasks. With practice, you'll soon be dressing your baby in no time, calming him in seconds, and changing his diapers in your sleep. While doing these basic tasks for your baby, you'll also develop patience, the ability to multitask, and the resourcefulness needed to amuse a baby during his umpteenth diaper change.

These tasks give you the chance to bond with your baby. While bathing and diapering him hold him, make plenty of eye contact with him, sing him special songs, and play silly games with him. Rocking him to sleep can be one of the most blissful activities of your day. Soon you'll find that doing these tasks lets you experience the joys of parenthood.

At the end of this chapter, parents who will eventually return to work can learn how to find reliable, competent day care for their baby.

Healthy babies aren't as fragile as you may think. Don't be afraid to touch, hold, rock, and cuddle your baby as often as possible. And don't let the soft spots (fontanels) on his head prevent you from holding, stroking, and caressing him. The thick membranes covering them are designed to protect his head until the skull bones fuse. You may notice pulsing veins under the skin of the soft spots—don't worry; that's normal.

Holding Your Baby

Holding your baby gives him physical and emotional security and aids his development. Touching and talking to him will make you comfortable with each other, so don't worry about spoiling your child by holding him whenever possible. (Besides, you can't spoil a newborn because every "demand" he makes is really a need, not a want.) Here are the best ways to hold your baby:

Option 1: Cradled in your arms.

Option 2: With your baby's head nestled against your shoulder while you support his back with one hand and his bottom with the other.

Option 3: Carrying him as you would a football. Lay your baby on his back along one of your arms, close to your side, and cradle his head with your hand.

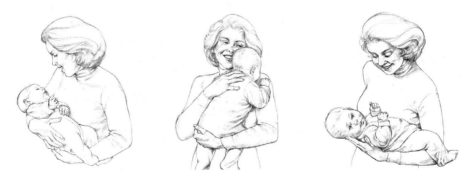

Picking Up Your Baby

During the first three or four months, it's important to support your baby's head when you pick him up and lay him down. He can't support his own head; his neck is too weak and his head is too heavy. Also, if you pick him up slowly and gently, you're less likely to startle him.

Option 1: If he's lying on his back, slide one hand under his neck and spread your fingers to cradle his head. Bend at the waist so you can comfortably slide your other arm under him. Lift him slowly in a compact bundle. Don't let his arms and legs dangle.

Option 2: If he's lying on his stomach, put one arm under his shoulder and neck. Cup his chin with your hand. Slide your other arm under his middle and spread your fingers to support his belly and thighs. Lift him slowly in a compact bundle. Or it may be easier to roll your baby gently onto his back and follow the instructions in option one to pick him up.

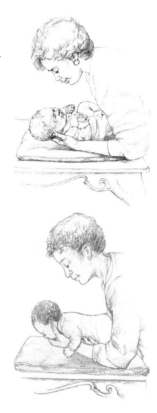

Note: It's okay for babies to be on their stomachs while they're awake and supervised. In fact, having some "tummy time" every day is important because it encourages a baby's neck and upper-body muscle development. But to help prevent sudden infant death syndrome (SIDS), the American Academy of Pediatrics (AAP) recommends that babies *always* sleep on their backs. (See page 46.)

To put down your baby: Lower his head and back while keeping your arms under him. Make sure you support his head. Lower his bottom, then gently slide both your arms from underneath his body.

Swaddling and Rocking

For the first month or two, most babies like being snugly wrapped in a receiving blanket, shawl, or wrapper-type sleep sack. Swaddling provides warmth and resembles the sensation of being in the womb. It can help calm a baby, help promote sleep, and it's a particularly good way to soothe a colicky infant (see pages 164–65), especially when you combine it with rocking. Rocking re-creates the motion your baby felt while in the womb. Don't rock too slowly; about sixty rocks per minute is a good pace. As they grow, babies eventually won't like to be swaddled and will prefer to move freely. Usually around two months, or when your baby tries to initiate rolling over, swaddling is no longer appropriate.

There are some risks to swaddling as well as benefits. By swaddling, your baby's arousal may be decreased, making it harder for him to wake up. There is some concern this may increase the risk of SIDS. For this same concern, a swaddled baby must always be put on his back. It is important not to overheat your baby when you swaddle him. If the swaddling is done too loosely, the blanket may become loose and pose a suffocation risk. Also, it is very important that your baby's hips are not wrapped tightly (such as in a papoose style), as this may increase the risk of hip dysplasia.

If your baby is taken care of by a day care provider before two to three months of age, you may want to discuss with the provider his or her practices on swaddling. Ideally, there should be continuity between what is done at home and at day care. But most importantly, the precautions just reviewed should be followed by the day care provider as well as yourself.

There are several ways to swaddle your baby. Excellent videos on methods of swaddling (referred to as "hip healthy swaddling") are available at the International Hip Dysplasia website at http://www.hipdysplasia.org/developmental-dysplasia-of-the-hip /hip-healthy-swaddling/.

The following instructions are for the "diamond" method of swaddling. The "square" method and a method that uses a commercial product called a sleep sack are other options demonstrated on http://www.hipdysplasia.org.

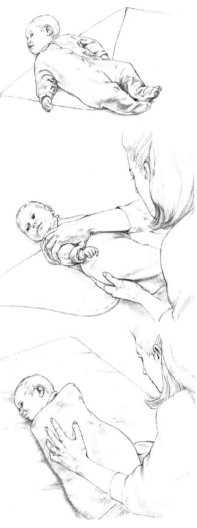

Step 1: Set a square blanket in front of you so it looks like a diamond. Fold down the top point so that the folded corner comes almost to the middle of the blanket. Lay your baby on his back on the blanket so his head is just above the fold.

Step 2: Straighten the left arm along the chest and wrap the left corner of the blanket over the body and tuck the blanket between the right arm and the right side of the body.

Step 3: Tuck the right arm down and fold the right corner of the blanket over the body and under the left side.

Step 4: Fold or twist the bottom of the blanket loosely and tuck it under one side, making sure that his legs are bent and his hips are open and can move freely (to prevent hip dysplasia).

Step 5: Make sure the blanket is not too tight. You should be able to get two to three fingers between his chest and the blanket.

A Note about Shaking Your Baby

Shaking a baby so his head jerks back and forth rapidly can break his blood vessels and cause irreversible brain damage. If you feel angry or frustrated with your baby, never shake him. Take a deep breath and count to ten, or ask someone to watch him until you can regain control. If you're alone with your baby, put him in a safe place (like his crib) and leave the room for a few minutes to calm down. For more information on this issue, see page 49.

Elimination

Changing diapers will probably never be your favorite task. Diapers leak and can stain clothing. Your baby may even pee on you in the middle of a diaper change. These things will happen, so keep your sense of humor and try not to make comments such as, "Yuck!" Your baby can't control his peeing and pooping (and won't for at least a couple of years), so showing your disapproval or disgust may send him the message he's done something wrong. Remember that the passage of urine and stool is an important indicator that things are going in well at the input end.

Urination

The Early Weeks

Don't be surprised if your newborn seems to always have a wet diaper. It's normal for a newborn to pee within twenty-four hours from birth and then up to thirty times a day. If your newborn stays dry for four to six hours or longer, call his health care provider. The darker your baby's urine color, the more concentrated it is. Dark-yellow urine can signify that your baby is not getting enough to drink. A baby's urine can also have a salmon-colored or pinkish tinge to it (referred to as "brick dust" urine). This is not blood but rather urate crystals, which also can suggest dehydration. Urinating should never be painful. If it ever seems that your baby is uncomfortable, have your care provider examine him.

The First Year

Starting from the third or fourth day after birth, your baby should wet at least six to eight diapers a day. If he wets fewer, make sure he's getting enough liquid. If he's breastfed, nurse him more often. If he's formula fed, it's okay to supplement his formula with water (no more than four ounces per day) in very warm weather. If he still isn't wetting enough diapers, have his care provider examine him. He may be dehydrated (see page 172).

Bowel Movements

Right after Birth

A greenish-black tar-like substance called meconium builds up in a baby's intestines before he's born. After birth, he'll poop out the meconium, usually beginning within the first day and continuing over the next one to two days, before normal digestion can start. Next to appear are browner, pastier stools referred to as "transitional" stools. The subsequent type of stool varies depending on whether your baby is breast or formula fed.

The Early Weeks

As your baby adjusts to feeding from the breast or bottle, his digestive system learns to function outside the womb. At first, he'll poop pretty frequently (and sometimes quite explosively), probably after every feeding or even more often. His stools will be loose and seedy or curd-like, and the color may vary. As long as your baby is feeding well and seems content, all these features are normal and don't suggest that he has diarrhea. (See pages 174–75 for more on diarrhea.) By the time he's three weeks old, his stools will have predictable characteristics, and he may poop less frequently.

Red, white, or black stools aren't considered normal. Consult your baby's care provider if his stools are any of these colors.

The First Year

- The breastfed baby: A breastfed baby's stools are usually mild smelling, mustard yellow, and loose. They may be greenish or brownish and appear seedy or watery; if they do, there isn't a problem with his digestion as long as he seems otherwise healthy. Because breast milk is so perfectly suited to your baby, it's almost impossible for him to become constipated as long as he's breastfed exclusively.

  Be aware that constipation refers to stool consistency only, not frequency (that is, how hard and difficult they are to pass, not how often they are passed; see pages 166–67 for more on constipation). After the first month, don't worry if he doesn't poop for several days. Even if he strains a bit when he finally does, the poop should be soft. Some babies poop several times a day, others, one time every several days. Both situations are normal, and it's also normal for babies to adjust their pooping patterns often. As long as your baby is thriving, there's no need to worry.

- The formula-fed baby: Because formula is less digestible and creates more waste than breast milk, the consistency of a formula-fed baby's stools is more solid than a breastfed baby's. The stools are usually brown or gold with a texture that resembles peanut butter, and they often smell like normal adult stools. A formula-fed baby can poop as often as six times a day early on, but then taper off to once a day (and sometimes once every few days) as he grows. If a formula doesn't agree with your baby, you'll probably first notice irritability and perhaps a change in his stools' consistency.

- At six months old, when solids are introduced: Any solid food that's new to your baby's digestive system may change the smell of his stools, and it may change their color to match the color of the new food (orange stools after eating carrots, for example). In older babies, undigested food may appear in the stools.

Diapers and Other Necessities

Disposable Diapers

Disposable diapers have a breathable outer liner, a core layer with absorbent gel that traps moisture into the middle, and a soft layer next to the baby's skin that keeps moisture away. Some disposables add lotion to help protect the baby's skin. Disposables have tab fasteners and elastic around the legs and waist to further prevent leaks. Have a good supply on hand when you bring home your newborn, because you'll probably use between 150 and 200 the first month. (Buy a few different brands to start; you'll want to compare them to learn which works best for you and your baby.)

Cloth Diapers

Nearly all cloth diapers are made of cotton, hemp, bamboo, or microfiber (some may include a bit of polyester). Cloth diapers let moisture evaporate and air circulate freely, allowing your baby's body to cool when heat builds. They usually come prefolded (with an additional more absorbent center strip) or fitted. Although not as popular as prefolded, flat diapers can be folded in different ways to fit your baby as he grows. Moisture-resistant diaper wraps cover the diaper snugly, and Velcro or snaps fasten most of them. Pull-on diaper wraps are usually looser; they require the diaper to be fastened by snaps, clips, or pins. All-in-one cloth diapers come with the diaper covers attached. If you use cloth diapers exclusively, you'll need two to three dozen diapers and three to six diaper wraps.

Hybrid Diapers

Hybrid diapers typically have a reusable moisture-resistant diaper wrap (similar to a cloth diaper wrap) and a disposable inner liner (similar to the core and inner layer of a disposable diaper).

Changing Area

You'll change your baby's diaper thousands of times before he's toilet trained, so it's important to have a safe, comfortable, organized place for this task. Here are some options for a changing area:

- Changing table: Check that it's sturdy and has a high guardrail, secure safety straps, and a place to store diapers, wipes, and creams. (Open shelves are more convenient than small, high-sided baskets, but make sure the shelves are out of reach of crawling or walking children.) Be wary of ones with flip-open changing areas that extend beyond the main table. The table may topple when a baby is placed near the edge of the overhang.
- Combination dresser and changing table: Again, be wary of ones with flip-open changing areas that extend beyond the main dresser. The dresser may topple when a baby is placed near the edge of the overhang.

- Wall-mounted fold-out changing table: This space saver attaches to the wall of your nursery or bathroom. They can be used for babies up to thirty pounds. Check for stability and secure safety straps.

- Play yard changing area: This removable pad attaches to the rails of a play yard. Check for stability and secure safety straps.

- Contoured changing pad: This thick, waterproof pad comes with safety straps and screws for attachment to a standard changing table. It also can be placed on the floor, dresser top, or elsewhere. If you use it on an elevated surface, make sure the surface is wide, sturdy, and a comfortable height. If you are using an elevated surface *other* than a standard changing table (like a dresser or bathroom counter), you can't anchor the changing pad to the surface; be sure the surface is nonslip.

- Portable changing pads: Typically used on the go, these waterproof fabric squares or fold-up nylon, vinyl, or plastic changing kits also can be used at home. They're best used on the floor, since they usually don't come with safety straps.

Diaper Wipes, Creams, and Powders

- Store-bought, disposable baby wipes are convenient but expensive. They're fine to use as long as they don't irritate your baby's skin (avoid those with alcohol or fragrance). A cheaper option is to clean your baby with a washcloth or soft paper towels and warm water.

- Some parents use a wipe warmer, a heated tub that holds and heats disposable wipes. This isn't a necessity, but your baby may enjoy it.

- Purchase a diaper barrier cream for everyday use. If your baby gets diaper rash, you'll also need a rash cream or ointment (see page 173).

- If you use a powder, make sure it doesn't contain talcum, which can damage your baby's lungs if inhaled. If you use any powder, shake it onto your hands, then apply to your baby's bottom; don't shake it directly onto your baby's bottom.

Diaper Pails

- If you use a diaper service, they'll likely supply you with a hamper that's lined with heavyweight plastic and includes a professional-quality deodorant.

- If laundering your own cloth diapers, you can use a plastic wastebasket with a flip-up lid, lined with a waterproof nylon laundry bag.

- For disposables, you may want to use a diaper disposer that compacts and deodorizes the diapers. Otherwise, a plastic wastebasket with a flip-up lid will work.

Choosing Diaper Care

Here's a quick look at the advantages and disadvantages of the four main options for diaper care: laundering cloth diapers, using a diaper service, using disposable diapers, and hybrid diapers. What option you choose will depend on a number of factors, including your schedule, your budget, your feelings about the environment and natural resources, and of course your baby's reaction to various kinds of diapers. Don't hesitate to search for cost-saving options including coupons and club savings.

Method	Advantages	Disadvantages
Laundering cloth diapers	• Requires no toxic chemicals; some laundries use toxic chemicals (such as phosphates, bleach) that leave chemical residues that can irritate baby's skin • Requires water and energy to launder, but less than are used in the manufacture of disposables • Is often the least expensive option of the three	• Is time consuming • Cloth diapers must be stored until laundered. • Few day care providers will use cloth diapers. • Can be inconvenient when you're traveling
Using a diaper service	• Saves time over laundering your own • Requires no rinsing or soaking • Is less expensive than using disposables • Diapers are laundered in accredited and inspected laundries, so you know diapers are clean.	• Is more expensive than laundering your own diapers • Is inconvenient when you're away from home • It may be hard to locate a service in some areas. • Some laundries use toxic chemicals (such as phosphates, bleach) that leave chemical residues that can irritate baby's skin.
Using disposable diapers	• Disposable diapers are ready to use from the package. • They can be tossed in any garbage receptacle (after contents have been flushed down the toilet). • Most day care providers insist on disposables. • They are very absorbent.	• Is usually the most expensive option • Infrequent changes, perfumes, and other chemicals may contribute to diaper rash and allergic reactions. • Disposable diapers require large amounts of wood, plastics, energy, and water to manufacture; they fill up landfills and take hundreds of years to decompose.
Using hybrid diapers	• Many can be used with either biodegradable disposable inserts or washable cloth inserts. • Many of the disposable inserts can be flushed down a toilet, or composted (if wet only). • Is a flexible system for parents who want an eco-friendly cloth system but sometimes need the convenience of disposable diapers	• Day care providers may not use them. • Can be inconvenient when you're traveling • Is more expensive than disposable diapers, unless you use the cloth inserts most of the time

Note: Some parents choose less common options, like "green" disposables or a diaper-free method called "elimination communication." For information on the former, check out manufacturers such as Seventh Generation (http://www.seventh generation.com) and Tushies (http://www.tushies.com). For info on the latter, see http://www.diaperfreebaby.org.

Diaper Care

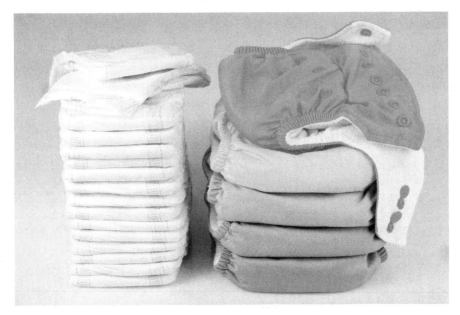

Obviously, cloth diapers require more care than disposables, if you wash your own. But laundering cloth diapers doesn't have to be time consuming or complicated (see the following laundering suggestions). If you use a diaper service, you won't have any diaper care. Simply empty the contents in the toilet, then toss the soiled diaper (no rinsing or soaking required) in the supplied hamper that's lined with heavyweight plastic and includes a professional-quality deodorant. A driver will regularly pick up the soiled diapers and leave you clean ones.

Soaking Cloth Diapers

Some parents prefer to presoak cloth diapers before laundering them to help reduce stains. They toss the soiled diapers into a diaper pail or washing machine with cold water and a cleaning agent (usually baking soda, vinegar, or borax), then let them soak for several hours or overnight. Other parents find soaking diapers unnecessary, especially if they use disposable diaper liners to protect the cloth. Some parents figure that diapers don't need to be spotless—they are, after all, *diapers*!

Laundering Cloth Diapers

There are various methods for laundering cloth diapers, but here's a particularly easy, effective routine:

1. Set up a dry diaper pail (a plastic wastebasket with a flip-up lid, lined with a waterproof nylon laundry bag), and toss in the soiled diapers. Keep the lid closed to contain odors.

2. Run the diapers through one cold-water rinse cycle (without detergent), then one hot wash cycle using a detergent (without bleach, which disintegrates fabric; or fabric softener, which ruins absorbency; or perfume, which may irritate baby's skin). Wash diaper wraps during that same hot cycle.

3. Machine dry the diapers or hang them outside to dry. (Sunshine will bleach them naturally.) If line-dried diapers are stiff, toss them in the dryer and run the air-fluff cycle for a few minutes.

4. To dry the diaper wraps, lay them on top of the dryer while the diapers are drying inside, machine dry them on the air-fluff cycle, or line dry them. (Don't machine dry them in a hot dryer; this may ruin them.)

Disposable Diapers

To get rid of a disposable diaper, dump as much of its contents into the toilet as possible. Then roll up and fasten the diaper in a compact bundle and toss it in the garbage, a diaper pail, or a diaper disposer that compacts and deodorizes the diapers.

Hybrid Diapers

Hybrid outer shells will need to be laundered, as will the reusable liners (see laundering instructions for cloth diapers above). The disposable liners can be tossed into the garbage (after dumping much of its contents into the toilet), flushed down the toilet (see manufacturer's instructions first), or, if wet, composted.

Diapering Your Baby

Tips

- Change your baby's diaper whenever he has pooped or is fairly wet. Don't feel as though you must change him if he's just slightly wet. Babies pee a lot, and you'll drive yourself crazy if you try to change him every time you detect wetness. As it is, you'll change ten to twelve diapers a day.
- Your baby may have a tendency to pee once the diaper area is exposed to air, so be prepared by keeping the open area covered.
- Unless your baby has an especially bad case of diaper rash, you don't have to change his diapers during the night. If he's sleeping peacefully and is covered, a wet diaper won't chill him.
- See page 173 to learn how to treat diaper rash.
- If you're using cloth diapers and your baby pees a lot while he's asleep, double-diaper him (fasten one diaper over another) before putting him down so you don't have to wake him for a change.
- While your baby's navel heals, fold the front edge of the diaper below the navel so it won't chafe and irritate the tender area. Some newborn diapers are cut out in the area of the navel to keep it from contact.
- Always keep a hand on your baby while he's on an elevated changing area. Even a newborn can wiggle to an edge and fall off.
- If you must leave the room in the middle of a diaper change, take your baby with you or lay him in a crib or other safe place.

Materials

- Diapers
- Soft washcloths with warm water, or disposable baby wipes
- Diaper barrier cream for everyday use
- Diaper rash cream or ointment

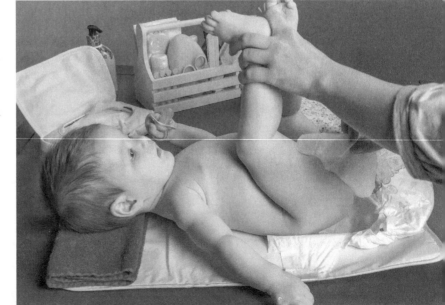

Step-by-Step

Step 1: Place your baby on his back on a changing area. Unfasten the diaper and remove it. If the diaper is soiled, roll it up and empty it into the toilet later. With a clean end of the diaper, wipe away any remaining poop from your baby's bottom. To help save your changing pad from accidents, you may want to place the clean diaper under your baby before removing the soiled one.

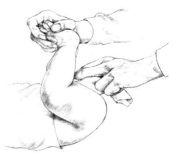

Step 2: Holding your baby's legs, lift his bottom and clean it with a warm washcloth or baby wipe, always wiping from his front to his back. Let your baby's bottom air-dry. Apply a diaper barrier cream. If he has diaper rash, apply diaper rash cream or ointment.

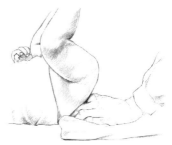

Step 3: Lift his bottom again and place the fresh diaper beneath (if you didn't do so in step 1), with the top edge of the diaper at waist level. With disposable diapers, make sure the tabs are behind your baby. With cloth diapers, fold over any extra material in front for a boy or in back for a girl. With boys, you may want to make sure the penis is pointed downward to prevent spraying out the top front of the diaper.

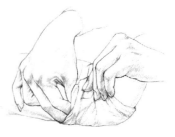

Step 4: After you cover the front of your baby with the front of the diaper, bring the tabs from the back of the diaper up over the front of the diaper, then fasten them securely at each side. Make sure the back overlaps the front. Check around the legs to make sure the ruffled area outside the elastic is not tucked in. If you're using pins with cloth diapers, put your hand between the diaper and your baby's skin to avoid sticking him.

Sponge Bathing Your Baby

Tips

- When your baby first arrives home, give him sponge baths. Don't bathe him in a tub until his umbilical cord has fallen off and the navel has fully healed. Also, if he's been circumcised, wait until his penis has completely healed before giving him a tub bath.
- You don't have to bathe or shampoo your child every day. As long as you keep his face, hands, and genitals clean, two or three baths a week is often enough.
- Newborns sometimes don't like being completely naked. If being naked annoys your baby, wrap him in a soft towel (unclothed or with just a diaper on) and uncover one part of his body at a time to wash it. Or leave him clothed, and remove clothing only when you want to wash the skin beneath it.
- Some newborns don't like to lie still long enough for a complete sponge bath. If your baby squirms, try bathing a different part of him throughout the day; for example, wash a different part each time you change his diaper.

Materials

- Bowl of warm water (test the temperature with your elbow, since it is more sensitive to temperature than your hand)
- Soft washcloths and a soft towel
- Cotton balls
- Mild, unscented soap (do not use "antibacterial" soap)
- Gentle baby lotion (optional—some advise no lotions for the first month, to prevent allergic reactions), or natural oil
- Sponge cushion (optional) or a large absorbent towel

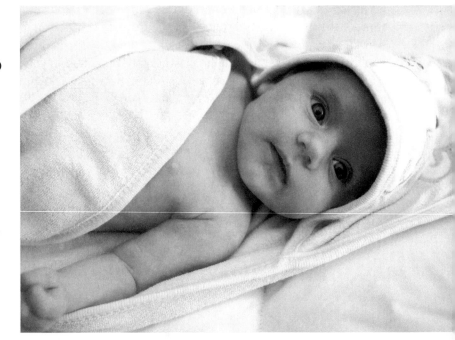

Step-by-Step

Step 1: Place your baby on a sponge cushion, large absorbent towel, or changing area. Moisten a cotton ball with warm water and wipe from the inside of one closed eye to the outside. Do the same to the other closed eye with a fresh cotton ball. Moisten another cotton ball and wipe around your baby's ears. Dampen a washcloth and clean around his mouth, chin, and neck.

Step 2: Hold your baby's head over a bowl of warm water and gently wet his scalp using the washcloth. Shampoo with a mild soap, massaging gently with your fingertips, not your fingernails. (Gentle rubbing can help prevent cradle cap—see page 168.) Rinse his head with the washcloth and pat it dry with a towel.

Step 3: Still using the washcloth, gently wash his chest, arms, and legs. Make sure to get into all the creases in his skin, including those around his neck and under his arms and knees. Wipe his hands and feet; check for lint between his fingers and toes. Also look for long or sharp fingernails and toenails. (See page 42 to learn how to trim nails.)

Step 4: Support your baby's head and gently turn him on his side. Wash and rinse his back. Pat it dry. Dampen a fresh washcloth and wash the genitals. For a girl, spread the labia and gently wash the skin from front to back, then pat it dry. For a boy, gently wash the penis and scrotum, getting into the surrounding creases. Wash carefully around a circumcised penis. If the penis is not circumcised, don't retract the foreskin to wash it.

Step 5: Check the navel for redness or swelling (signs of infection). Know, though, that it's normal for the base of the cord to ooze and stink a bit as it dries up. If your baby's skin is prone to dryness, warm some gentle baby lotion or natural oil in your hands and massage it into his skin. Put a fresh diaper and a fresh outfit on him, and your baby's sponge bath is done.

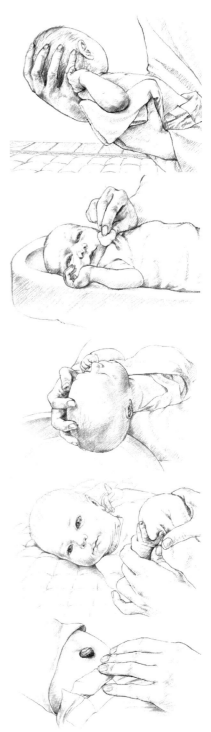

Tub Bathing Your Baby

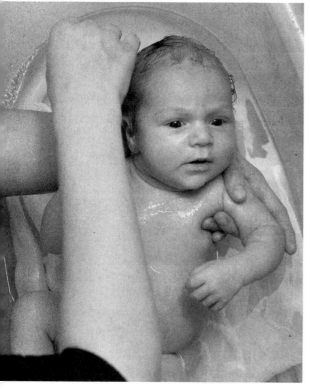

Small Tubs

Tips

- At first, your baby might not like taking baths. Continue giving him sponge baths until he's a little older, then try giving him a tub bath. Eventually, most babies love taking tub baths.

- As with sponge baths, you don't need to bathe or shampoo your baby every day. As long as you keep his face, hands, and genitals clean, two or three baths a week is often enough.

- Never take your eyes off your baby while he's in the tub, no matter how short a time and how little water you're using. If you must interrupt the bath to answer the door or phone (for example), quickly wrap him in a towel and take him with you.

- Be careful: babies are slippery when they are wet.

Materials

- Portable baby tub with sponge cushion (A plastic dish tub will work for a smaller baby. You can also bathe your baby in the kitchen sink as long as you can rotate the faucet away from the sink.)
- Table or countertop at a convenient height
- Soft washcloths and a soft towel
- Mild, unscented soap (do not use "antibacterial" soap)
- Baby shampoo
- Gentle baby lotion (optional—some advise no lotions for the first month, to prevent allergic reactions) or natural oil

The Big Tub

- When your baby is too big for his baby tub and he can sit up steadily on his own, he's probably ready to bathe in a regular bathtub.
- Run only a few inches of water in the tub to reduce the risk of drowning or even unintentional dunking. *Never leave your baby unattended in the bath.*
- Always test the bathwater before putting your baby in the tub. It should feel pleasantly warm. Keep him away from the faucets; one turn of the hot water tap and he could scald himself. After drawing the bath, run a little cold water so the faucet won't burn your baby if he touches it.
- At first, you may want to bathe with your child so you can better keep a hand on him. (This way, you also don't have to kneel on a hard floor and bend over throughout his bath.) Later on, you can place nonslip strips on the bottom of the tub to help keep your baby steady.
- When your baby can stand, don't let him do so in the tub without keeping a hand on him.

Step-by-Step

Step 1: Run about two inches (5 centimeters) of warm water in the tub, then check the water temperature to make sure it's pleasantly warm. Extreme temperatures can scald, burn, or shock an infant. Gently ease your baby into the tub, bottom first.

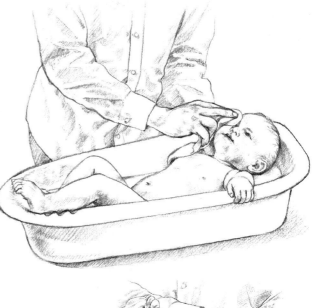

Step 2: Wash your baby's face, ears, and neck with a soft washcloth and gentle soap. Work your way down his body, washing him just as you would with a sponge bath. (See pages 36–37.) Rinse well.

Step 3: Support your baby in a reclining position and shampoo his head, working from front to back so the shampoo doesn't get into his eyes. Rub the scalp firmly but gently with your fingertips. Rinse well, then pat him dry with a soft towel.

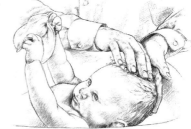

Skin Care

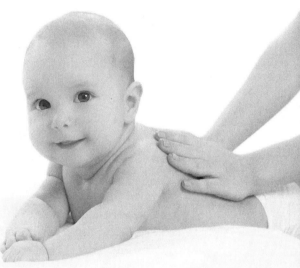

An occasional bath is all the skin care your baby needs. Some parents apply powders and lotions to make their babies smell good and keep the skin from drying out or chafing. These products aren't necessary (and some care providers advise against their use in the first month); the best way to avoid dry skin is to not bathe your baby too often. In general, use skin care products sparingly and heed the following warnings:

- Baby (talcum) powders and cornstarch: Baby powder can get into your baby's lungs, swelling and irritating them and possibly causing breathing problems. It can also inflame the skin affected by a diaper rash. Some research suggests that cornstarch can cause or exacerbate yeast infections.

- Baby lotions and natural oils: While these products aren't needed, your baby may love being gently massaged with a little lotion or oil after his bath. (See page 41.) You may want to apply any oil or lotion you use to a small area of skin first to make sure no rash develops.

Navel

Before your baby's umbilical cord stump falls off, make sure you keep the area clean and dry. Give him sponge baths only, and make sure his diaper is turned down away from the area. You don't need to clean the area with rubbing alcohol; in fact, many hospitals no longer recommend this treatment.

The stump usually falls off between one and three weeks after birth. (If it doesn't fall off by three weeks, have your baby's care provider examine it.) When it does, it leaves a raw spot that can take several days (or even weeks) to heal. There's no need to bandage the area. Keep it clean and dry to prevent infection. A little secretion or pinkish discharge from the navel is normal, but tell your baby's care provider if there's any bloody discharge that continues for more than a week, any profuse bleeding, or any red swelling. Sometimes the cord will continue to ooze a moist yellow discharge. This is caused by an umbilical granuloma; it usually can be treated in the care provider's office with a silver nitrate cautery stick. If this doesn't work, the care provider may use surgical thread to remove it.

Penis
Circumcised
The tip of the penis will be red and swollen up to a week after circumcision. A yellow or gray coating may appear on the tip of the penis where the foreskin was cut. If a scab is present, let it fall off on its own. It's normal for the wound to ooze a few drops of blood. Until it's completely healed (usually within a few days but possibly up to a week), wash the tip by dripping warm water on it, then pat it dry. When you change your baby's diaper and after every bath, dab the tip with a barrier jelly or place a piece of gauze smeared with barrier jelly on it. Once it's healed, you can wash it normally and can stop using the jelly.

Contact your baby's care provider if you notice any of these warning signs:
- Your baby doesn't pee normally within six to eight hours after the circumcision.
- The tip of the penis is persistently swollen, bleeding, or red.
- The tip leaks foul-smelling fluid or develops crusted, fluid-filled sores.

Uncircumcised
The uncircumcised penis requires no special care. Wash it as you would any other part of your baby's body. Don't try to retract the foreskin; the head of the penis doesn't need cleaning. Natural secretions clean it very efficiently. These white secretions aren't dirt or pus; they're healthy skin debris that will eventually separate the foreskin from the head by the time your child's five or six years old (but possibly not until adolescence).

As with any other part of his body, contact your baby's care provider if the penis and foreskin is very discolored, emitting an unusual discharge, or bleeding.

Vagina
There may be some blood passed through your baby's vagina in the first few weeks. These "mini-periods" are from maternal hormones and will go away on their own. It is not necessary to wash away all of the whitish secretions that accumulate in the folds of the vaginal tissue.

Baby Massage
Babies are especially sensitive to touch, so your baby may find a light, gentle massage extremely soothing and comforting. You can massage a little baby lotion or natural oil into your baby's skin after his bath. (Set the bottle in his bathwater to warm the lotion or oil.) Slowly, gently, and rhythmically massage his neck, then massage down his body to his feet. Don't forget his arms and hands. Turn him over and massage his shoulders, back, and buttocks. Finally, massage his forehead and down his face. Many hospitals and community centers offer classes on baby massage.

Trimming Fingernails and Toenails

Keeping your newborn's fingernails and toenails short protects him—and you! As he explores with his hands and feet, long and ragged nails can scratch his face and body as well as yours. Short fingernails are also a health precaution; dirt collects under long fingernails, and it'll be years before your baby quits putting his fingers in his mouth.

Here's what to do when you cut your baby's nails:

- Use baby nail clippers. Make sure there's enough light to see what you're doing. Before clipping, press the skin away from the nail to avoid clipping the fingertip.
- Trim the fingernails or toenails when your baby is asleep or after a bath, when his nails are softer and easier to cut.
- Cut fingernails and toenails straight across. Make sure you leave no ragged edges.

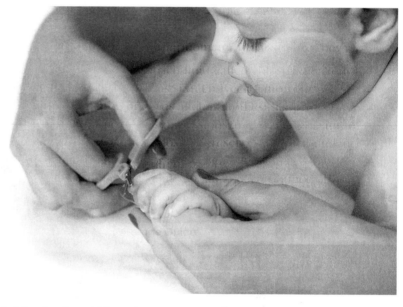

If you do clip a fingertip, don't worry. Nearly every parent does it at least once. Wrap a facial tissue around your baby's finger and hold it above his heart. The bleeding will likely stop in a couple of minutes. If it takes longer than that, your child is probably still okay. Put him someplace safe where you won't mind some possible bloodstains. Although putting on a bandage seems logical, try not to do so, especially on a fingertip. Bandages can easily come off fingers and toes and can become choking hazards to babies.

Sleep

Functioning on less sleep is one of the biggest adjustments parents of newborns have to make. As your baby grows during the first year, he'll sleep through the night more often, which means you will, too. But it may take a few years before your sleeping is back to its prebaby schedule.

Sleep needs and habits vary among babies. The average newborn sleeps between sixteen and seventeen hours a day, but often only one to two hours at a time. (Keep in mind that newborns usually need to feed every two to four hours around the clock.)

Even though you may think he sleeps too little or too much, he's probably getting enough if he's healthy. You probably can't resist checking on your baby as he sleeps, especially if you hear his snuffling and fretting. Don't let these normal noises alarm you.

As the first year progresses, your baby may take a couple of naps during the day, then sleep for a stretch of time at night. (See page 47 to learn more about sleeping through the night.) Not long after his first birthday, he may even give up one nap. The older your baby gets, the more active he'll be during the day, especially when he starts crawling and walking. And the more energy he expends during the day, the easier he may fall asleep at night.

Bed Options

Your newborn will need a safe place to sleep. There are many advantages to having your baby sleep in the same room as you, a practice called co-sleeping. Research suggests that co-sleeping promotes bonding and breastfeeding and helps prevent sudden infant death syndrome (SIDS).

It is not recommended for babies to sleep in the same bed as parents (bed sharing), as this increases the risk of SIDS and accidental smothering. There is also a risk of the baby falling, or getting wedged between the bed and the wall or headboard. Thus the practice of room sharing but not bed sharing has the most advantages.

Beds

- Bassinet or cradle: Both are compact, but bassinets are typically portable; your baby will outgrow both of them quickly. Babies about one month old or ten pounds will usually need a crib.
- Crib: Once you are finished with using a bassinet or cradle (if you have one), a crib can be your child's bed until age two or older. (See page 119 for what to look for in a crib.)
- Play yard: This convenient, portable product is great for travel because it can be used as a crib, bassinet, changing table, and play area.

Bedding

- Mattress for crib, bassinet, or cradle: Use a firm, nonallergenic mattress, because a soft mattress can suffocate a baby. (An innerspring mattress will hold its shape longer than a foam mattress.)
- Waterproof mattress pads: You'll want one or two of these pads to place between the mattress and the fitted sheet.
- Fitted sheets for crib, bassinet, or cradle: Make sure the sheet fits tightly and securely around the mattress.
- Bumper pads: Bumpers should not be used because they can suffocate your baby (and can be used as steps to climb out).
- Blankets, pillows, and soft toys: These are also suffocation hazards and should not be used.
- Do not use wedges to elevate your baby's upper body.
- Mobile: A windup mobile can soothe baby to sleep, but make sure it meets safety standards. The mobile needs to be removed as soon as he can push himself up.

Environment

- If your baby's bed isn't in your bedroom, begin a routine of putting him to sleep in his bedroom. He'll gradually connect the routine with sleep time and settle down. Plus, if he's sleeping in another room, his restless sleep periods won't distract you.
- Keep the temperature of your baby's room around 70°F (21°C). A room that's warmer than 70°F may overheat the baby and possibly lead to SIDS. If you're trying to conserve energy or cut your heating bills, turn your thermostat down at night and put your baby in a blanket sleeper. (*Don't* use an electric blanket or space heater.) Putting your baby by an interior wall may also keep his temperature more consistent.
- Besides overheated environments, other factors that can lead to SIDS and suffocation, entrapment, or asphyxia are soft or loose bedding and bed sharing, especially on sofas, soft mattresses, or waterbeds or with parents who have consumed drugs or alcohol before going to bed or who smoke while in bed.
- Immunize your baby. This also decreases the chance of SIDS.
- When necessary, use a cool-mist humidifier or vaporizer in winter and a fan in summer, but don't set them too close to your baby's bed. Follow the manufacturer's guidelines to clean the humidifier or vaporizer so it won't contaminate the air with molds. Also, use the purest water you can so any waterborne contaminants won't be spread.
- Your entire household doesn't need to keep silent while your baby sleeps. He'll easily get used to the normal sound levels. Try to avoid, however, abrupt changes in the noise level, which can startle and awaken him.
- To block outside light as well as summer heat and winter cold, install shades or curtains in your baby's bedroom.

- In comfortably warm weather, your baby can take naps outside, but don't put him in direct sunlight. Drape netting over his bed to ward off insects.
- Always place your baby on his back to sleep to reduce the risk of SIDS.
- Never cover his head while he's sleeping.
- Do not use a car seat as a place to put your baby to sleep.
- Do not use commercial devices that claim to promote prevention of SIDS, like a wedge positioner or a wearable monitor. They have not been proven to reduce SIDS, but putting items into your baby's crib has been proven to increase the incidence of SIDS.
- The American Academy of Pediatrics (AAP) currently does *not* recommend that babies younger than six months share a bed with parents.

Getting Your Baby to Sleep

Newborns seem to have three kinds of sleep:

- Quiet sleep (deep and calm)
- Active sleep (accompanied by sucking, grimacing, and rapid eye movements)
- Drifting sleep (drowsily floating in and out of sleep)

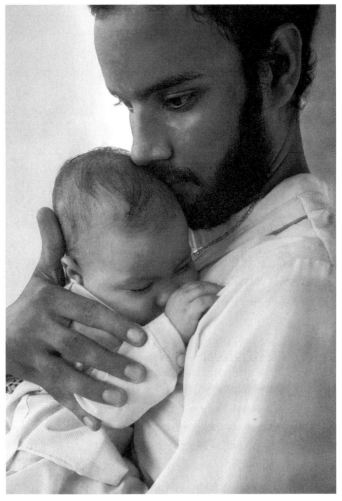

Early in his first year, your baby may need help falling asleep. A newborn often has trouble learning to shut out outside stimuli. The best way to help settle your baby down so he can prepare for sleep is to soothe him. Some breastfed babies may be helped by non-nutritive sucking. Using a pacifier can help calm your baby as well as help decrease the chance of SIDS. Never tie a pacifier—or anything else with a cord or string of any kind—around his neck. If he is hungry, nurse him or give him a bottle. Do not wake your baby for a feeding unless you have been given instructions to do so because he's had poor weight gain or infrequent urination or stooling. Never give him a bottle to feed or soothe himself in the crib. If he's not hungry, try the following ideas:

- Swaddle or rock him until he falls asleep. When he's four months old or so, set him in his bed before he's completely asleep so he learns to drop off by himself.
- Car rides, stroller rides, swings, and holding him as you walk will often lull an excited baby to sleep.
- Use soft, rhythmic background noise. Soft music will work, but so will the drone of a fan, vaporizer, dishwasher, or air conditioner. If you play a recorded heartbeat over and over right after birth, it may remind your baby of life in the womb and calm him. Place the music player or white noise machine across the room and at a low volume to prevent causing any possible hearing problems.
- Lay your baby across your lap on his belly and give him a gentle back rub.
- Fresh air often makes babies sleepy. Take your baby outside for a while, or put his bed at a safe distance near an open window if it's not too chilly.

Make sure your baby gets plenty of physical activity, stimulation, and one-on-one time during the day; some parents find this helps baby sleep better at night. Remember the motto Daytime Is Playtime. Pay attention to signs he shows that he is getting sleepy.

Sleep Positions

The American Academy of Pediatrics (AAP) recommends that babies sleep on their backs. Research shows this sleeping position significantly reduces the risk of sudden infant death syndrome (SIDS). (The risk of your baby choking on spit-up or vomit while sleeping on his back is minimal.)

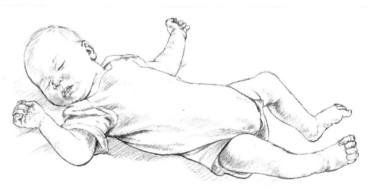

You should make sure grandparents and all other caregivers know the importance of this position for sleep (this is a fairly recent safety change, but a very important one). Statistics show SIDS has been decreased by 50 percent as a result of placing babies on their backs to sleep.

Staying Awake at Night

Babies don't know that they're supposed to sleep at night and be awake during the day. Some sleep more during the day, which usually means these babies are wide awake and ready to play at 4 a.m.! Here are some things you can try to get your baby sleeping at night:

- Try not to let him sleep more than three or four uninterrupted hours during the day.
- Stimulate him during the day by singing or massaging him. But at night, be quiet and calm while attending to him, and keep the room dark.

Sleeping through the Night

Some babies seem to master sleeping through the night from very early on, and others seem to struggle endlessly with it. Breastfed babies may wake more frequently than bottle-fed babies; the milk is digested more rapidly so they become hungry sooner than a bottle-fed baby. A baby who is a healthy sleeper is not necessarily a baby who sleeps deeply all night but one who can settle himself back to sleep on his own.

Parents often wonder what to do when their baby wakes at night. As your baby gets older, it is good to wait a few minutes and see if he will fall back to sleep on his own. Eventually, he should be able to be put down for bed when he is still awake.

Two behavior-modification techniques may be helpful if your older infant is struggling with sleep. "Controlled comforting" is a method in which a parent responds to a cry at increasingly longer intervals to help allow the baby to settle himself. "Camping out" involves a parent sitting in the sleep room and then quietly retreating as the child learns to fall asleep independently.

Comforting a Crying Baby

One challenge for new parents is to figure out why their baby is crying and how to stop it. In itself, crying is an important way for babies to communicate. It is normal for newborns to cry between one to four hours a day. It is especially common for babies to have a fussy time in the early evening hours. It may be possible to recognize different types of cries (e.g., a hunger cry can be very different from a cry of pain). Pay attention to not just if but *how* your baby cries, as you may be able to better direct how you help him. Most times you can comfort your baby by satisfying a basic need—feeding him, changing his diaper, entertaining him. The following paragraphs describe reasons why a baby may cry and offer some suggestions for comforting him.

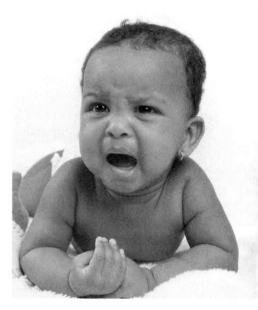

Hunger

Often a crying baby is a hungry baby. Crying is his last resort to get someone to feed him. Babies give earlier, calmer cues to show they're hungry, like sucking on a fist or rooting (see page 21), and it's wise for parents to respond to these cues. Food may be what a crying baby wants, but it can be difficult to feed him when he's upset.

Gas in Stomach

To burp your baby, use one of the techniques described on page 97. Some babies need one burp for every three to five minutes of feeding. Some babies are delayed burpers; a half hour may pass from the end of a feeding to the first burp. If your baby is a delayed burper, be patient and keep trying. He'll eventually pass that gas!

Need to Suck

Most babies are born with an intense sucking reflex. They suck not only to get nourishment but also to soothe and comfort themselves (referred to as non-nutritive sucking). If you're nursing your child, the breast is the best source of comfort for him. But if he's clearly not hungry, help him find his (clean) fingers to suck or offer one of your own. Don't give him a pacifier frequently for the first few weeks; sucking on it may interfere with his latch on your breast. If your baby is bottle fed, go ahead and give him a pacifier.

Wet or Soiled Diapers

As you can imagine, having a wet, stinky mess next to your skin is uncomfortable. On average, newborns wet or soil ten to twelve diapers each day. If your baby is cranky, he really may be demanding a diaper change. (Even if a diaper change doesn't stop his crying, at least it's reduced the chances he'll acquire a diaper rash.)

Temperature Extremes

Babies, like adults, don't like to be too hot or too cold. Don't overdress your baby, leave him in drafts, or take him out into cold weather if he's not properly bundled. Dress him as you would to keep yourself comfortable in any environment.

Boredom

Babies, like adults, can become bored. Your baby's crying may be his way of requesting some stimuli. (See pages 133–36 for ways to entertain a bored baby.)

Overstimulation

A baby's senses can get overloaded if there's *too much* stimulation. Loud noises, bright lights, and crowds in particular can overwhelm your baby, causing him to cry. Placing him in a dim, quiet room should solve the problem. Otherwise, background or white noise (e.g., from a vacuum) may help calm your baby. Never place your baby on top of a clothes dryer to comfort him; he could fall off.

Inadequate Physical Contact

Newborns need lots of physical contact with their parents and other caregivers, and they'll cry if they don't get enough. Remember: It's impossible to hold, stroke, or caress your baby too much. Placing your baby in a front carrier or sling is a great way to keep your baby close to you while keeping your hands free.

Colic

Many babies younger than three or four months have a fussy period almost each day or for several hours at a time when nothing seems to comfort them. If your baby fits this description, he may have colic. See pages 164–65 to learn more about colic and find suggestions for coping with it.

Warning about Shaking Your Baby

Although you may become frustrated by your baby's crying or irritability, *never* shake your baby. Serious injuries (including blindness, brain damage, and abnormal development) occur when a baby is severely or violently shaken or when his head is struck. This represents a serious form of child abuse. A baby suffering from non-accidental head trauma (or NAHT, also called shaken baby syndrome) may vomit, have tremors, convulsions, or breathing trouble, and become very listless or fussy or even comatose as a result of the injuries. It's urgent that you seek immediate medical attention for your baby if there is any chance that he's suffering injuries from shaking or being hit in the head. If you're worried that you might be capable of losing control when your baby is crying or irritable, put him down in a safe place such as his crib and let him cry alone. Take a deep breath and count to ten. Seek help from family and friends to give yourself a break, and have your baby's care provider examine him to see if there's a reason he's irritable.

Non-Nutritive Sucking

Sucking lets a baby soothe himself (non-nutritive sucking) or get nourishment. When your baby is fussy and you know he isn't hungry or in need of a diaper change, having him suck on his thumb or fingers or on a pacifier (but only if breastfeeding is well established) may calm him.

According to the American Dental Association (ADA), non-nutritive sucking won't harm the development of a baby's teeth or mouth if the sucking isn't too frequent or intense, but prolonged sucking (past four years), and frequent, intense sucking may cause dental problems. Most children give up non-nutritive sucking when they're between two and four years old, but they may revert to the habit if they're tired, stressed, or afraid. This is a natural reaction and isn't a reason for concern.

Thumb and Finger Sucking

If your baby prefers to suck on his fingers or thumb, try to always keep them clean. If your baby is upset and doesn't naturally suck on his fingers or thumb, you can gently guide it to his mouth and see if he'll take it and calm down.

Pacifiers

Pacifiers may reduce the incidence of SIDS, but this does not mean you need to try to force your baby to take a pacifier. If you are breastfeeding, do not introduce a pacifier until breastfeeding is well established; a pacifier can make early breastfeeding difficult, because sucking on it may interfere with how a newborn latches onto the breast. Some parents and experts find that pacifier use is an easier habit to break than thumb or finger sucking.

Here's some advice about pacifier use:

- Make sure the pacifier is in one piece and has a soft nipple. (Don't use the nipples from bottles. Alone, they're too small to be safe. Even when attached to a ring collar, a bottle nipple may be pulled loose by strong sucking.)
- Check that the shield is at least one and a half inches (3.8 centimeters) across and is made of firm plastic with air holes.
- Make sure the pacifier is the right size for your child. (Pacifiers come in two sizes: one for the first six months and one for older children.)
- Check that the pacifier doesn't have ribbons attached to it. (Tying a pacifier to a crib or to your child poses the risk of strangulation.)
- Replace the pacifier when the rubber has changed color or become torn.
- Don't pop a pacifier in your baby's mouth whenever he's fussy. First make sure he doesn't need something else: food, dry clothes, warmth, cuddling, or whatever.
- If your baby needs to suck a pacifier to fall asleep, he'll probably wake up and cry when it falls out of his mouth. To solve this problem, try to remove the pacifier when he gets sleepy.
- Never sweeten a pacifier; doing so can cause tooth decay. (Babies under a year of age should never be given honey because of possible botulism poisoning.)

Clothing and Shoes for Your Baby

Clothing

Babies grow quickly during the first year, so don't be surprised if your baby rapidly out-grows his clothes. On average, babies double their birth weight in four to six months and triple it by the end of the year. Babies also generally grow eight inches (20.3 centimeters) during their first year.

Baby clothes can be expensive, and it's hard to get your money's worth when your baby is growing like a weed and staining everything in sight. Following are some strategies for stretching your baby's clothing budget:

- Borrow clothing from friends and family.
- Use saved clothing worn by your other children (and save clothing worn by this baby for any future children).
- Buy smart:
  - Buy baby clothes at consignment or thrift stores and garage sales, where you'll often find high-quality, gently used items at great prices.
  - Buy clothes on sale or at outlet stores.
  - Buy big, and keep shrinkage from washing in mind when you buy.
  - Choose multipiece outfits; they provide more flexibility. Larger pieces of the outfit can still be worn when smaller pieces do not fit.
  - Buy clothes that allow for simple adjustments as baby grows larger: clothing that can be let out by snaps, straps, buckles, and cuffs.
  - Cut the feet out of stretchies and have baby wear booties.
  - Look for fabrics that give, like terry cloth and knits.

Unfortunately, baby clothing manufacturers don't adhere to a standard sizing system. Some companies use the labels *small, medium, large,* and so on; others label their clothes by months of age, still others by weight. To make matters worse, the same term can mean different things to different manufacturers. When shopping for baby clothes, look for clothes labeled by weight, or take your baby with you so you can eyeball items for proper fit. If neither of these strategies is possible, use one of the following charts to help you choose clothes that will (hopefully) fit your baby.

Size	Height	Weight
General		
X-Small	Up to 24 in.	Up to 12 lb.
Small	25 to 26 in.	13 to 17 lb.
Medium	27 to 29 in.	18 to 22 lb.
Large	30 to 32 in.	23 to 26 lb.
X-Large	33 to 37 in.	27 to 30 lb.

Size	Height	Weight
By Age		
Preemie	Up to 18 in.	Up to 6 lb.
Newborn	17 to 21 in.	6 to 8 lb.
0 to 3 mos.	20 to 24 in.	7 to 12 lb.
6 mos.	24 to 27 in.	12 to 16 lb.
9 mos.	27 to 29 in.	16 to 18 lb.
12 mos.	29 to 31 in.	18 to 23 lb.
18 mos.	31 to 33 in.	23 to 26 lb.
24 mos.	33 to 35 in.	26 to 29 lb.

Look for the following features when buying, reusing, or borrowing baby clothing. These features will better ensure the clothes are practical, safe, and comfortable for your baby.

Practical Features
- Long wrist and ankle cuffs to accommodate growing limbs
- Full cut, extra limb length, and/or adjustable snaps for growing room
- Front opening, crotch opening, and/or encased elastic for easy dressing, undressing, and diapering
- Minimal fasteners that are easy to manipulate
- One-piece design for speedy change of outfit
- Machine washable and dryable fabric, with colorfast dye, including trim
- Wrinkle-free fabric
- Sturdy construction
- Accessories (such as matching bibs, vests, hats, or blankets) usable after baby has outgrown other parts of outfit
- Gender-neutral design that can be handed down to a baby brother or sister

Safety Features
- No drawstrings, toggles, straps, sashes, or belts that hang loosely and pose strangulation hazards
- Roomy but not-too-loose fit (Loose-fitting coats and oversize or baggy clothing can get caught on furniture, in doors, and so on.)
- Naturally flame-retardant fabric (like polyester or fleece) or snug fit for fire safety: If your baby must wear clothing that isn't flame retardant, make sure it fits snugly so there's little air between the fabric and your baby's skin. (Air feeds a flame if the fabric is on fire.)

- No bows, buttons, appliqués, or other trim to prevent choking (or make sure they are securely fastened; check every time)
- No loose threads that could entangle baby's fingers or toes and cut off circulation
- Generous neck, arm, and leg openings for easy breathing and circulation
- Clearly identified manufacturer in case of questions, complaints, or recall

Comfort Features
- Seams flat, smooth, and minimal in number
- Minimal or no trim
- Collars, buttons, bows, appliqués, snaps, and/or seams are soft, nonbulky, and located where baby won't be lying on them
- Fit that's not too loose or too tight
- Soft, breathable fabric
- No features on inside of clothing (embroidery backing, zippers, stiff tags, and so on) that might irritate baby's skin

Keeping Your Baby Cool or Warm

Babies can have a difficult time maintaining their body temperatures. They produce heat from birth but need time to develop the ability to conserve that heat. Until he learns to regulate his internal thermostat, here are some tips for dressing your baby so he's at a comfortable temperature:

- In cold weather, dress your baby in layers so you can add or take off clothes as the temperature warrants. For a newborn, a short trip in cold weather is usually fine if he's bundled properly. For a longer trip, your baby may become chilled, especially if he falls asleep. Also, make sure his cheeks aren't exposed for a long time; they get cold quickly.
- In warm weather, parents often mistakenly overdress their baby. Overdressing can cause rashes and dehydration through excess sweating. When you're out of an air-conditioned environment, dress your baby in as little clothing as possible and keep him out of the sun.

Dressing Your Baby

As your baby grows and becomes more active, he's not likely to keep still while you dress him. With practice, you'll learn how to wrangle him into an outfit. But you'll probably also rely on games and songs to keep him quiet and perhaps a special toy to keep him amused.

- To put on a shirt, gather the neck opening into a loop. Slip it first over the back of your baby's head, then forward. Stretch the opening as you bring it down gently past the forehead and nose so you don't scratch his face.

- To pull on sleeves, put one of your hands through the wrist opening and up the sleeve, then grab your baby's hand. With your other hand, pull the sleeve over his arm.
- To take off a shirt, take your baby's arms out of the sleeves first, then stretch out the neckline. Lift the neckline over the nose and forehead, then slip the shirt off toward the back of the head.
- To put on a one-piece outfit, start by spreading it out on a flat surface, then laying your baby on top of the outfit. Slide his legs in first, then his arms, and zip or snap it closed.

Shoes and Socks

Before your baby walks, he doesn't need shoes (except to protect his feet on rough or hard surfaces and for warmth). Even when he starts walking, bare feet will help him master the task faster. Babies are born with relatively flat arches. By walking on his bare feet, your baby builds up his arches and strengthens his ankles. Plus, he can use his bare toes for balance. When you decide your baby needs shoes, here are some things to keep in mind:

- A baby just learning to stand may have trouble balancing while wearing shoes. He may fall often until he gets used to them.
- For walking on uncarpeted floors, avoid socks or booties that don't have slip-resistant soles.
- To ensure a good fit, take your baby along when you buy him shoes. Measure the width and length of his feet, then look for shoes that match those measurements. Check the size of your baby's shoes every three months.
- Try on shoes with the appropriate socks for the season. Socks should also fit well. (If they're too small, they can constrict your baby's toes.)
- Have your baby stand or walk in the shoes to see how they fit. There should be a half inch (1.25 centimeters) of space beyond his longest toe to allow for growth.
- Baby shoes can be expensive, but you don't need to buy the priciest, sturdiest shoes. As long as they fit well and your baby's comfortable wearing them, a pair of inexpensive shoes will work.

Clothing Checklist

Following are the kinds of clothing your baby most likely will wear during the first year. You might not need all of the items, and what and how many items you'll need will depend on how often you do laundry, the season, and your baby's age, among other factors.

Item	How Many	Description
Soft cotton shirts	4–7	These shirts provide extra warmth when worn under other clothing. In warm weather, your baby may be comfortable wearing just a shirt and a diaper.
Onesies	4–8	These one-piece cotton bodysuits that snap at the bottom make dressing your baby easy.
Bodysuits and overalls	6	These one-piece suits cover your baby from neck to toe and can be worn day or night. The front snaps make it easy to change them, and the stretchy material is comfortable and allows room for growth. Overalls are practical and comfortable for older babies who are starting to creep or crawl.
Dresses		In general, dresses aren't practical for babies. If you want your baby to wear a dress, choose shorter ones. Longer dresses tend to get in a crawling baby's way.
One-piece pajamas	4–7	One-piece pajamas are like coveralls made of soft material that's great for sleeping. Avoid those that have plastic on the bottoms of the feet; these can make your baby's feet sweat.
Sleep sacks with or without swaddling wrap	2–4	A sleep sack is like a cozy sleeping bag for your baby, except it's fitted over his shoulders and has cutouts for his arms. Unlike pajamas with feet, a sleep sack can come off and go back on quickly for easy diaper changes. Some sleep sacks come with a wrap piece attached that swaddles your baby.
Socks or booties	4–7	These are used only for keeping your baby's feet warm in cooler temperatures. Babies' feet are naturally cool, so let the temperature guide whether your baby needs them.
Food bibs	4	Some bibs slip over your baby's head, and some fasten around the neck. Some even have long sleeves that will help keep his clothes clean. Some plastic ones have a pocket at the bottom designed to catch falling food.
Caps, bonnets, or hats	1–3	Cotton or synthetic caps or wide-brimmed bonnets work well in warm weather to protect your baby's head and face from direct sunlight. Knitted hats will keep your baby's head and ears warm in cool or cold weather.
Sweater or jacket	1	Sweaters are available in front- or back-opening styles. (Wool sweaters are scratchy and can be a pain to launder. Plus, some babies are allergic to wool.)
Snowsuit (or one-piece fleecewear)	1	Snowsuits are made of heavy, durable material. Many have optional snap-on mittens and hoods. Choose one that's a little big because it'll have to cover your baby's clothes. They're great for outings in cooler weather. Thick snowsuits should not be used in a car seat; instead dress your baby in warm clothes, and cover the car seat in warm blankets or a car seat cover.
Winter mittens	1 pair	Baby mittens are knit bags with drawstrings around the cuffs, making them easy to get on and off your baby's hands.
Receiving blankets	4	These soft, lightweight blankets can swaddle or cover a newborn; act as a changing area; and become extra padding when rolled up in a car seat.
Warmer blankets	2	Blankets are warm and washable. They wrap easily and stay tucked around your baby in a car seat or stroller. (Never use blankets in your baby's crib.)

Finding a Day Care Provider

The right child care for your baby depends on your family's needs. You may choose to stay at home and provide the care yourself. Or you may plan to return to work full time or part time and arrange for child care during your working hours.

Child care options include formal, licensed day care (day care center and home day care) or informal day care (nanny, au pair, care by a relative, or share care, in which two or more families share the cost of and care by a nanny). Each type of child care has advantages and disadvantages. You must weigh the pros and cons of each before choosing the child care that best ensures your baby's safety and well-being, meets your family's needs and budget, and gives you peace of mind.

If you decide to use a licensed day care center or home day care, follow these steps to find the best one for your baby. Be patient and prepared to visit many providers. This search may take a lot of time and energy, but don't settle for a less-than-perfect day care. Remember: Your baby deserves the best care you can find. (For information on babysitters, see pages 63–65.)

1. Know what you want. Are you looking for a day care near your home or your work? Do you want your baby around lots of other kids or just a few? How much can you afford to pay? Will you need a lot of flexibility?

2. Broadcast your search and research your options. Ask friends, family, health care providers, coworkers, and houses of worship to help you find the most reputable day cares. Some employers offer child care referral benefits; check with yours. Call the Child Care Aware hotline at 800-424-2246 to find the phone number of your local child care resource and referral agency, which can refer you to licensed and accredited centers and home day cares in your area, or go to their website at http://www .childcareaware.org. Check other online resources, too. Visit http://www.naeyc.org or http://www.nafcc.org to find day care guidelines and contact information. If all else fails, check with your local chamber of commerce or social media for day care centers and home day cares in your area. If a day care sounds promising to you, note its name and phone number, the name of the person who referred you, his or her evaluation of it, and what he or she paid for its services.

3. Visit and interview day cares. You can ask basic questions over the phone (for example, about fees and available openings), but you won't know what a day care is really like until you visit it. The more time you spend interviewing a potential day care provider, the better. At each interview, note the name of the day care, the name and position of the person you're interviewing, the day care's address and phone number, and the date. Trust your intuition and pay close attention to how the center's staff or the home day care provider answers the questions on pages 57–61. After the interview, ask for a copy of policies and a schedule of the day's activities, then record your observations and impressions of the day care.

4. Check references. Ask parents why they love a certain day care provider. Nothing provides a ringing endorsement of a day care like other parents' positive evaluations. Ask parents specific questions. Don't simply ask whether they *like* the day care; ask what exactly they like about the care and what they don't. Here are other good questions to ask:
    - How old are your kids, and how long have they been enrolled in the day care?
    - If your children are no longer enrolled, why did you remove them?
    - How did you select the day care?
    - How has the day care helped you with normal developmental issues and concerns?
    - Have you had any problems with the day care? How have you resolved differences?
    - Have your children ever been hurt in day care or not wanted to attend day care? What happened?
    - Have you had your children in other care? How do the day cares compare?
    - What's the best feature about the day care? Any weak points?

> **Background Checks**
> To find companies you can pay to do child abuse, criminal, driving, credit, and social security or work authorization background checks on potential day care providers, use the keywords *background check* in an online search. Another option is to check the Yellow Pages under *investigators* or *security*.

5. For added assurance, call your state's Better Business Bureau to find out whether any complaints have been filed against the day care.

6. Make an unscheduled visit. Dropping in unannounced can provide you with a more accurate picture of the day care's day-to-day operations. Does the care seem as excellent as it did during your formal visit?

7. Visit the day care with your child. See how he or she and the provider(s) interact. Does your child seem comfortable in the environment?

8. Get on the waiting list, if it's an option. If the perfect day care doesn't have space for your child, securing a spot on the waiting list nearly always means that your child will get in—eventually. In the meantime, ask the day care to recommend other similar places, and arrange for other care (share care, relative care, or other) until a spot becomes available.

Day Care Interview

Fundamentals and Philosophies
- When did the day care open for business?
- Is the day care licensed and inspected? Is the license current? Is the day care accredited?
- How many children are enrolled? What's the age range?
- Is there a separate room for infants? How many babies are in the room? Is the infant-to-provider ratio no more than three to one in a center or two to one for a home day care?
- Will the same person care for my baby every day?

- How does the provider stimulate babies throughout the day? Will my baby be kept in a swing or bouncer seat? For how long? Will my baby be allowed on the floor? Is the floor padded? Is the floor cleaned daily?

- What's the daily schedule of activities? Does it include outdoor play? Does it include TV viewing? If so, how much? Are there any circumstances where children leave the center or home and, if so, is there a transportation policy? Do the children have identification on them in case they get lost?

- How do the provider and any assistants respond to crying infants? How do they discipline disruptive children? What are some examples? How willing is the provider to follow my discipline guidelines?

- What is the provider turnover rate? What's the average term of employment?

- Will I be notified if a new provider takes over care of my baby? Can I request a particular provider?

- Who can I regularly talk to about my baby's development, behavior, and needs? Will my baby's activities be recorded daily? Can I review the log?

- Are visits (expected and unexpected) from parents welcome?

- What does the day care expect from parents? What is your policy on how you communicate with parents?

> **Separation Anxiety**
>
> At first, your baby might not mind being separated from you and having another person care for him. Once he's about seven months old, however, he may develop separation anxiety and stranger fear. If your baby doesn't want you to leave him in a new environment, try to make the transition gradual by not leaving him and walking away suddenly until he seems more at ease.

Provider Qualifications

- What are the providers' educational backgrounds, credentials, and training? How about interests, experience, or social affiliations?

- How are candidates screened?

- Do all employees undergo federal background checks, including criminal and child abuse checks?

- Must employees pass regular physical examinations and have up-to-date vaccinations?

- Are providers first-aid and CPR certified (including infant training)?

Health and Safety

- What's the day care's sick-child policy? What if the illness is minor? How will I be notified when my baby is ill?

- How often does the day care experience outbreaks of serious contagious illness? How will I be notified of an outbreak?

- Is there a qualified health professional, such as a doctor or nurse, for the program? (Day care centers should be visited every month; home day care should be visited every three months.)
- Does the day care require a physical examination before accepting a child?
- Does it accept children who aren't vaccinated?
- Has a child ever been seriously hurt while in the day care's care? What happened?
- Has anyone pulled a child out of the day care's care? If so, why?
- What is the policy on biting and other child-inflicted injuries?
- What's the protocol if the day care suspects a child is being hurt at home or school?
- How does the staff manage children with allergies or special needs?
- Will my child's medical records and emergency information be posted in plain sight? Will the staff dispense prescription medications? Where will medications be stored? How are they measured and dispensed?
- What security measures does the day care have in place? Does it have a sign-in and sign-out sheet? Are the entrances monitored? What's the policy for having someone other than a parent pick up a child?

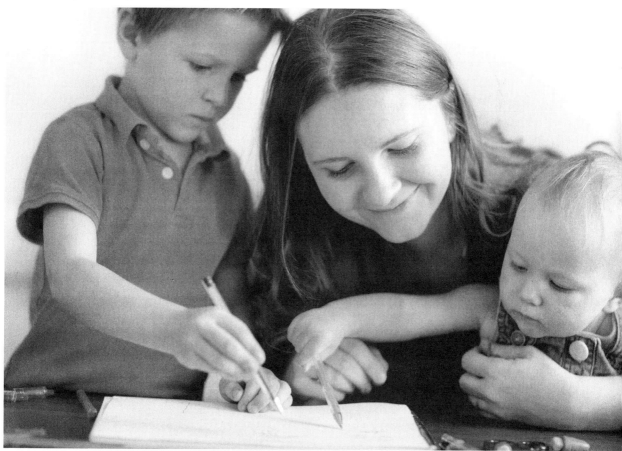

- Are firearms kept in the home or day care? If so, are they stored unloaded in a lock box or gun safe and out of children's reach?
- Are fire extinguishers and smoke and carbon monoxide detectors present and in working order? Where are the fire exits? Are monthly fire drills performed?
- What's the cleaning schedule?
- Are cleaning products toxic? If so, are they and other toxic substances locked out of children's reach?
- Are the food-preparation and diaper-changing areas sanitized frequently?
- How old are cribs, changing tables, and other equipment? How is the day care notified of product recalls?
- Will babies have their own cribs?
- How often are linens changed? How are they laundered?
- Does the staff make sure babies sleep on their backs, to help prevent SIDS?
- Does the day care have an enclosed play yard?
- Are the toys age appropriate? How old are they and how often are they cleaned and replaced?
- Are providers required to wash their hands after diapering and feeding each child?
- How often do they wash the children's hands?

Sleeping, Feeding, Diapering

- Will my baby be held during feeding?
- Can my baby be fed breast milk? How will breast milk be stored?
- Does the day care have a place for nursing moms to breastfeed? Am I able to come and breastfeed my baby at any time?
- Is there a feeding schedule? A napping schedule? Will my feelings about scheduling be respected?
- Does the day care provide meals and snacks or should I bring food for my child? What food is served?
- Where and how often are diapers changed? How are diapers disposed of?
- Is the day care willing to use cloth diapers?

Fees and Operation

- What are the day care's hours and holiday schedule?
- What's the policy for closing for inclement weather?
- What are the fees for babies? What are the fees for older children? How often are fees raised? Are there any additional fees? Will I be charged when I'm on vacation or my child is sick at home?
- Are pickup and drop-off times flexible?

- Will I be charged a late pickup fee? How much?
- How and when will I be billed?
- Will I need to provide supplies for my baby, like diapers and bottles?
- Will the day care advise me of child care tax credits and provide receipts?
- Is there an opening for my child? How do I apply?
- Is there a waiting list? How long a wait can I expect?
- Does the day care give preference to siblings, if I choose to have more children?

References

- May I have a list of families I can call for references? (Make sure the list contains both families currently enrolled in the day care and families no longer enrolled.)

Observations and Impressions

- Does the day care have definite rules and regulations, a firm sick-child policy, emergency backup care plan, and staff members with solid, current credentials?
- Are the providers' CPR and first-aid training adequate? Do they appear responsible, enthusiastic, and well prepared? Do they seem to share your philosophies on key parenting issues like sleep, discipline, and feeding?
- Is the provider-to-child ratio acceptable? (See sidebar on page 62.) Do the providers appear to care for the children without difficulty? Keep in mind that an acceptable ratio is compromised if toddlers are always in the infant room, or if one of the babies has special needs.
- Do the provider and children seem happy and engaged? Is the general mood joyful and playful?
- Are the children under constant, attentive supervision?
- Do the providers hold the babies? Talk and sing to them? Do they respond to crying babies immediately? When you ask them about individual children, do they seem to know each one and his or her needs and personality?
- Is the day care inviting and clean? Clutter-free and organized? Does it seem overcrowded?
- Are the rooms adequately heated, air-conditioned, ventilated, and lighted? Are the food preparation, eating, sleeping, and changing areas impeccably clean? How about the restrooms?
- Is the day care childproofed? (Open cupboards and crawl on the floor—your baby will.) Does the staff observe basic safety rules? Do you notice any safety problems like cords or tripping hazards? Do the crib sheets fit tightly (to reduce risk of sudden infant death syndrome, or SIDS)? Is the play area fenced in and away from streets?
- Is emergency information clearly posted? How about phone numbers for the police, fire department, and poison control? Where are the first-aid supplies located?

- Is the environment stimulating? Is the schedule of activities varied? Does TV play a minimal role?
- If the day care serves meals and snacks, are they nutritious?
- What's the noise level? Is the napping area quiet? Is there background music?
- Does each infant have his or her own crib and cubby space (for pacifiers and other personal items)?
- Do the children's charts appear current, complete, and packed with detailed entries?
- Does the provider seem willing to listen to your concerns and happy to answer your questions?
- Will you feel at ease knowing your child is in this setting?

Adult-to-Child Ratios

The ratio of adults to children can vary, depending on group size and state licensing requirements. (Contact your state's health and human services department to learn the adult-to-child ratios for your state.) The National Association for the Education of Young Children (NAEYC) has set these guidelines:

Day Care Centers

- For infants, the ratio is 1 adult for every 3 children if a group has 6 babies, 1 for every 4 if a group has 8 babies. Group size of 6 is recommended.
- For toddlers (age 12 to 24 months), the ratio is 1:3 for 6 children, 1:4 for 8 children, 1:5 for 10 children, and 1:4 for 12 children.
- For children (age 24 to 36 months), the ratio should be 1:4 for a group of 8 children, 1:5 for a group of 10, and 1:6 for a group of 12.

Centers aren't required to follow NAEYC's guidelines, so ask what each center's ratio is and decide whether it's okay for you. A good center will keep the groups of children small regardless of staff size.

Home Day Cares

The NAEYC recommends that a home day care provider should care for no more than 2 babies (under age 30 months), 5 preschoolers (age 30 months to 5 years), and 2 school-age children (age 5 or older) at once.

Babysitters

Whether you're planning to stay at home with your baby or you're returning to work and arranging for day care, it's vital to have an evening out alone every now and then. When you're ready to leave your baby in a babysitter's care, follow these steps to find the perfect one for your family.

Search Early

If possible, start searching for a babysitter before your baby arrives. Ask friends, neighbors, relatives, other parents, and day care providers whether they know of any good candidates. Call the student employment service at a local college or high school and post fliers at gyms, youth centers, places of worship, or post the inquiry on social media. A baby-sitting agency is a good source for finding prescreened sitters (check your Yellow Pages for more information). You'll have to pay the agency for its services, but agency employees are usually older and more experienced than average teenage babysitters.

Interview candidates. Once you have a list of candidates, look for someone you feel is old enough to do the job well. That person may be as young as age eleven, if he or she seems confident and knowledgeable about child care. Most parents feel comfortable with a babysitter who's older (usually no younger than age fourteen), and one who has gone through certification with first aid and CPR, but you're the best judge of a babysitter's ability to care for your child.

Ask each baby-sitting candidate the following questions. During the interview, trust your instincts and pay attention to how the candidate answers the questions. After the interview, if the candidate seems promising, introduce him or her to your baby. Watch how they interact and record your observations and impressions.

Babysitter Interview

- How long have you been babysitting?
- Do you have experience caring for infants? Are you trained to perform CPR and first aid (including infant training)?
- Why do you like working with children?
- What do you like best about babysitting? What do you like least?
- What other child care experience do you have?
- Do you still babysit for your prior clients?
- What are the ages of other children you've watched?

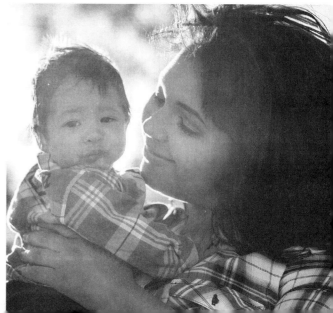

- What activities do you enjoy doing with children?
- How do you soothe a crying baby?
- What's the best way to put a baby down to sleep?
- Have you ever given a baby a bath?
- If the babysitter will be transporting your baby:
    - What kind of car do you have?
    - What's your driving record?
    - Do you know how to install and use a car seat?
- If the babysitter will be feeding your baby:
    - How do you prepare a bottle (breast milk or formula)?
- If you have pets:
    - Are you allergic to any animals?
    - Are you comfortable around pets?
- Do your parents support your baby-sitting jobs (if the babysitter is under age eighteen)? Will your parents be home while you're babysitting?
- What do you do in your spare time? Any hobbies? Other jobs?
- Tell me about your school life. Sports? Activities? Grades? Do you like school?
- Will you need a ride to and from your house?
- How much per hour do you charge?
- May I have a list of families I can call for references?

Call References

After you've selected a few promising candidates, it's important to call their references. Don't ask former employers whether they simply *liked* the babysitter; ask them the following specific questions and note their answers in detail:

- When and for how long did the babysitter work for you? How did you hire him or her?
- How many children do you have? What gender and how old were they? Any infants?
- What was your general impression of the babysitter? What did he or she do especially well? What tasks could he or she have done better? Anything you would change about him or her?
- How would you describe the babysitter's personality? Was he or she caring and warm? Patient? Respectful? Creative? Prompt and reliable? Did he or she have a positive attitude? Lots of energy? Sound judgment? Initiative?
- Did your children get along well with the babysitter?
- How did the babysitter handle emergencies? What's an example?
- How did the babysitter discipline your children? Did you ever suspect child abuse? Did you conduct any background checks?
- Was the babysitter clean and well groomed?

- Did the babysitter follow your rules and respect your home? Any problems with drinking, smoking, or unauthorized visitors?
- Would you use this babysitter again?
- Would you mind sharing pay information?
- Any advice on ways to develop a good working relationship with this person?
- Anything else I should know about him or her? May I contact you again if I have additional questions?

Prepare for Your Babysitter

Before leaving your baby in a babysitter's care for the first time, arrange for the babysitter to visit your home so he or she can get to know you, your home, and your baby. You can ask him or her to arrive a half hour or so before your scheduled departure. Or if you feel your babysitter doesn't have a lot of experience caring for infants, you may want to pay him or her to drop by and care for your baby a few times while you're home. You can use the time to take care of other tasks, knowing that if problems arise, you're nearby.

Give the babysitter as much information as you can, from emergency phone numbers (including the phone number of the place you'll be, and your cell phone number) to your baby's sleeping, feeding, and bathing schedules—even include what food is off limits. If your baby needs medication, show the babysitter how and when to give it to him. If you're going someplace where you can't be contacted, call home periodically and leave the phone number of someone the babysitter could contact in case of an emergency. (Make sure ahead of time that person will be home.) Have a flashlight and first-aid chart and supplies handy, and review your fire escape plan with the babysitter.

If your babysitter will be in your home for more than three hours, make sure there are snacks and meals for him or her to eat. And always be on time or communicate any changes.

Remind your babysitter to never leave your baby alone.

Maintain the Relationship

Once you've established a good relationship with a babysitter, it's important to maintain it. Trusting a babysitter with your baby should tell him or her a lot about how you feel about the relationship. The responsibility should make him or her want to do the best job possible. Tell your babysitter specifically what you've noticed that he or she does well. And always remember to treat your babysitter with respect. This may be his or her first real job, and he or she wants to be considered mature and capable.

Chapter Three

Feeding Your Baby

Feeding the baby is one of the greatest joys of early parenting. There's no more cherished feeling than providing your baby nourishment as she lies nestled warm and relaxed in your arms.

A baby grows more during her first year than at any other time in her life. Her weight generally triples by her first birthday, and she typically grows eight inches (20.3 centimeters) over her first twelve months. (See the weight and length charts on pages 220–21.) What your baby eats determines how well she'll grow.

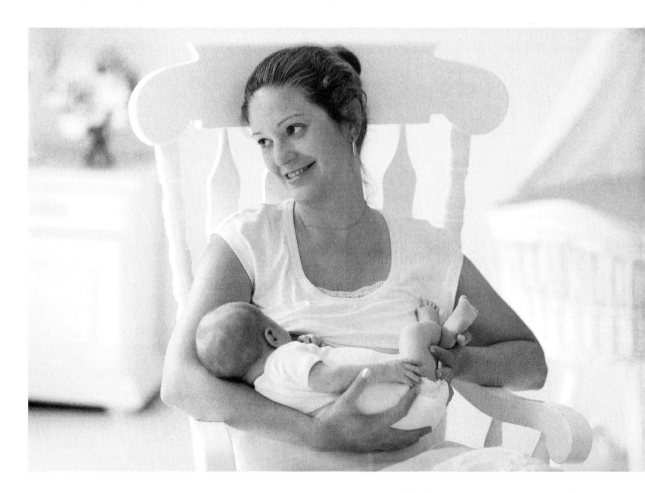

Research continues to affirm that breastfeeding is immensely important to babies, mothers, and society. The American Academy of Pediatrics (AAP), the American College of Obstetricians and Gynecologists (ACOG), the World Health Organization (WHO), and the US Preventive Services Task Force recommend that babies breastfeed for at least the first year of life. Furthermore, babies should ideally consume only breast milk for the first six months. These studies and recommendations have fueled a resurgence of breastfeeding in North America, which was a formula-feeding culture for several decades. The most recent statistics indicate at least 79 percent of new mothers try to breastfeed, with a goal by 2020 of 82 percent of mothers starting to breastfeed and 62 percent continuing at least some breastfeeding by six months of age.

To support initiation of successful breastfeeding, WHO and the United Nations Children's Emergency Fund (UNICEF) have named strict criteria and designated hospitals that meet the declared initiatives as official "Baby-Friendly" hospitals. To check the designation status of any hospitals you are considering for your delivery, go to https://www.babyfriendlyusa.org.

Breast milk meets a baby's nutritional needs perfectly, and no formula can match it. Plus, no bottle can exactly imitate the breast as the perfect way to deliver milk. If breastfeeding is impossible, however, formula provides adequate nutrition. And it's certainly true that there are formula-fed babies who are just as happy and healthy as breastfed babies. But the evidence strongly suggests breastfeeding betters the chances that a baby will enjoy great health, now and for the rest of her life.

To help you make the best choice for your family, the following list outlines the primary pros and cons of breastfeeding and formula feeding. You'll want to choose a feeding method well before your baby's birth. Both breastfeeding and formula feeding require some preparation and planning.

Breastfeeding and Formula Feeding: A Fact-Based Comparison

Breastfeeding

Pros
Infant

- Provides milk that's all natural and made specifically for your individual baby
- Adapts to baby's needs, which is especially important for premature or ill babies who require more calories and nutrients; breastfed premature babies have lower rates of infection than formula-fed premature babies.
- Provides optimum nutrition for baby; breast milk contains just the right amount of fatty acids (DHA and ARA), lactose (milk sugar), water, probiotics and prebiotics, and amino acids. These promote proper human digestion; brain, eye, and hearing development; plus, overall healthy development of baby.
- Provides baby with antibodies that help protect against infections of the ears, lungs, and gastrointestinal tract; newborns are born with immature immune systems that make these substances of special importance. Breastfed babies have fewer acute illnesses, including ear infections, even after breastfeeding is discontinued. They also have fewer physician visits and hospitalizations for illnesses.
- May help protect baby against allergy development; breast milk is an immunologically active substance, and breastfed babies have fewer wheezing episodes in the first two years of life than formula-fed babies. They may also have a lower risk of developing an allergy to cow's milk and a slightly lower risk of eczema.
- Likely helps protect baby against a number of terminal and debilitating diseases, like sudden infant death syndrome (SIDS), childhood leukemia and lymphoma, inflammatory bowel disease (Crohn's disease), meningitis, and diabetes
- Makes infants less stressed, based on their response to painful procedures, perhaps because of raised cortisol levels and increased maternal bonding
- Is easy to digest, which means less constipation, diarrhea, and gas in baby; results in less stinky spit-up and bowel movements
- Encourages baby's proper jaw and tooth development
- May have the potential to increase your baby's IQ

Mother

- Helps mom's uterus return to normal size by stimulating production of the hormone oxytocin

- Burns mom's calories (about five hundred per day), which can help facilitate maternal weight loss

- Is economical: Costs typically include a breast pump, bottles, nipples, nursing bras, and nursing pads; typical cost is $500 (depending on the type of pump purchased); money is also saved by having fewer indirect costs, like additional physician and hospital visits, time off work for illness, etc.

- Is convenient: Baby's nourishment is always on hand and ready to eat when mom and baby are together.

- Is environmentally sound: It requires no manufacturing or packaging and produces no waste.

- Is emotionally satisfying and enjoyable for mom and baby: It gives mom regular surges of the "happy, calming" hormones, prolactin and oxytocin.

- Enhances mother-baby bonding

- Typically makes traveling with baby easy

- Helps protect mom against ovarian and breast cancers; may decrease risk of type 2 diabetes, rheumatoid arthritis, and cardiovascular disease; appears to help protect mom against heart disease and osteoporosis

- Protects maternal iron stores because it delays menstruation

- Exclusive breastfeeding in the absence of menstruation can provide a natural form of contraception for up to six months; it is wisest, however, not to rely entirely on breastfeeding as a contraceptive.

- Ensures mom sits or lies down regularly to rest

Cons

- Must be learned: Though natural, breastfeeding is rarely "automatic." Mastering breast-feeding can be difficult in the first few days and weeks for both mom and baby. Make sure you get support and guidance from knowledgeable, empathetic support groups, professionals, and family and friends.

- May seem difficult if mom had a cesarean birth; cesareans can cause a delay in milk coming in, and the baby might press on mom's incision while feeding. With nurs-ing and pumping often, however, and with continued feeding attempts, mom's milk should come in. Also, mom can use different positions (such as lying down or the football hold) to keep her baby off her belly.

- May draw unwanted attention in public, but with a little practice, it's easy to breastfeed discreetly. With more and more women breastfeeding, the sight of a woman nursing in public is becoming more accepted. In addition, federal and state lawmakers are currently passing laws that support breastfeeding in public (and in the workplace).

- Some moms feel uncomfortable or anxious about breastfeeding because of earlier trauma, a lack of physical self-esteem, or simple modesty. Make sure you get support and guidance from knowledgeable, empathetic support groups, professionals, and family and friends.

- May cause mom physical discomfort, like cracked nipples and engorged breasts; try to prevent these problems through proper positioning, frequent feedings or pumping, and beneficial routines like breast massage and nipple-cream application.

- Only mom can breastfeed. Today's breast pumps allow mom to express and bottle breast milk anywhere easily and quickly, which lets others enjoy feeding baby mother's milk and lets mom maintain her milk supply.

- May make it hard to tell how much the baby has eaten; if the baby is wetting four to six disposable (or six to eight cloth) diapers and soiling three to four diapers in twenty-four hours, then she is probably consuming an adequate amount of breast milk.

- Breast milk does not contain an adequate supply of vitamin D. While regular exposure to sunlight should be enough, many breastfed babies will need to be given a supplement.

- Preparing the breast milk for day care takes more work, and some day care providers will not use breast milk. Start pumping extra breast milk as soon as you are able to, and check with day care providers when you initially interview them.

There are times, despite all efforts, that breastfeeding just doesn't work or, rarely, isn't advised (if the mother is too ill and/or in need of certain medications—your health care provider will let you know if this is the case). If you've done your best and can't breastfeed, don't worry. Your baby will get adequate nutrition through formula feeding, and you can still bond by holding her close during feedings.

Formula Feeding

Pros
- Provides adequate infant nutrition when mother's milk is unavailable (if mom is absent or ill) or when the baby is unable to metabolize or digest it (if she has a rare condition such as galactosemia)
- Can be fed to baby by anyone without mom's involvement
- Anxiety or modesty about your body is not a factor.
- Easier for day care: Typically you just need to provide a can of powder and a couple of clean bottles.
- Flexibility if mom needs to be away, is sick, or needs sleep
- Mom's diet is not a factor.

Cons

- Is nutritionally inferior to breast milk; today's formula is still missing about a hundred nutritional components found in breast milk.

- Provides no antibodies

- Can't be guaranteed safe; contamination may occur at the manufacturing plant.

- Can be time consuming and inconvenient; toting bottles, preparing and heating formula, and washing nipples and bottles takes a lot of planning and time.

- Raises baby's risk of illness; formula-fed babies are ten to fifteen times more likely to become hospitalized when ill.

- Is expensive: The average American family spends approximately $1,500 a year to formula feed a baby. This amount includes the cost of the formula, bottles, and nipples.

- Doesn't help mom's postpartum physical recovery

- Does not promote the transfer of "happy, calming" hormones, prolactin and oxytocin, from mother to child through breast milk; also, affords less direct skin-to-skin contact, which is soothing to baby and good for mom

Breastfeeding Basics

Physical Preparations

Your pregnant body will naturally prepare your breasts for breastfeeding. Early in pregnancy, your areolas (the base of the nipples) darken. Your breasts enlarge, and your body stores extra fat throughout the pregnancy for the energy it'll need for breastfeeding.

Here are some things you can do to prepare your body for breastfeeding:

- Wash your nipples with water only, not soap. Soap can wash away natural protective oils.
- Don't use lotions and ointments on your nipples unless instructed to. They can clog pores and cause irritation.
- Wear a well-fitted bra to help prevent future sagging. You can even wear adjustable nursing bras before delivery.
- If you've had breast cancer or breast surgery, especially breast reduction surgery or nipple transplantation, consult a breastfeeding specialist and your surgeon about whether you can breastfeed. You will want to find out if the milk ducts or major nerves were affected by your surgery.
- If you have had your nipples pierced, there is a chance that latching on will be difficult, but help and support from specialists should allow you to succeed.
- Don't "toughen" your nipples. Aggressive nipple tweaking may damage the tiny glands in the areola and in late pregnancy could release a hormone that starts labor contractions. (Gentle tweaking—during sex, for example—is fine.)
- If your nipples are inverted, talk with your care provider about breastfeeding. He or she will help you decide if you need to take steps during your pregnancy to prepare your nipples.
- Keep in mind that the size of your breasts has absolutely nothing to do with your ability to nurse. Milk is produced in glands deep within the chest; the fatty tissue that makes breasts doesn't influence milk production in any way.

Emotional and Mental Preparations

While your body prepares physically for breastfeeding, you can prepare mentally and emotionally. First and foremost, it's important to have a positive attitude. Breastfeeding can be difficult at times, and your postpartum hormones may make your mood changes more severe, so be sure to avoid naysayers and seek support systems that will help you initiate and maintain successful nursing. Ask your care provider or childbirth educator about breastfeeding classes in your area and available lactation consultants (breastfeeding experts who are trained to care for breastfeeding mothers and babies). You can also contact your local La Leche League or the International Lactation Consultant Association (http://www.ilca.org) for breastfeeding support.

First Feeding

Ideally, your baby should be given to you for skin-to-skin contact immediately so you can begin to breastfeed (if you are not able to start immediately, then within the first hour preferably). Breastfeeding immediately after birth has been shown to increase overall success in breastfeeding, not only the initial latch on but long-term success. Any unnecessary interventions (like taking the baby's weight) should be postponed if possible to allow for this priority. Babies are in an alert stage immediately after birth, followed by a sleepy stage for several hours. Your baby should "room in" or stay with you as much as possible while you're at the hospital or birth center. Make your breastfeeding plans and wishes very clear to the birthing staff.

If you have a cesarean section or difficult delivery, the first feeding may be delayed but should still be attempted in the delivery room if possible.

Colostrum

At first your breasts produce a thin, yellowish, nutrient-rich fluid called colostrum. (You can express colostrum by squeezing the areola as early as sixteen weeks into your pregnancy.) This substance is packed with nourishing proteins and antibodies that protect babies from harmful infections. Early and frequent nursing sessions are very important to ensure that the breasts will eventually produce milk. Colostrum reserves aren't abundant, and you may worry that your baby isn't getting much for all her nursing. Don't worry; a newborn's stomach is the size of a walnut, and it takes only about a quarter ounce of colostrum to fill it up. Don't supplement her feeding with formula unless her care provider or a lactation consultant recommends it.

Transitional and Mature Milk

Your breasts start producing milk usually two days (if this isn't your first baby) to six days (if this is your first baby) after giving birth. If you've had a caesarean section, your milk may come in later than after a vaginal delivery. (In this case, keep trying to feed your baby and consult with her care provider or a lactation consultant.) The milk gradually transitions from colostrum to mature milk. How much milk you produce changes to meet your baby's needs. Breast milk looks a lot like skim cow's milk (thin, clear, white), but unlike skim milk it will separate if stored in the refrigerator. (Gently swirl the milk to mix it.)

Successful Latch

A baby's sucking is a reflex. (See page 21.) Latching on refers to the formation of a tight seal of the infant's lips around the nipple and the correct amount of breast. Latching on to a breast and suckling might not come as naturally to some babies. These babies must learn how to position themselves correctly on the breast, grip, suck, and swallow while nursing. If a baby frequently sucks on an artificial nipple or a pacifier in the first three weeks, she may have trouble latching on properly for nursing (this is called nipple confusion). A correct latch shouldn't be painful (although at first you may feel some pain for about a minute), should stimulate a healthy milk supply, make milk flow better, keep your baby content, and prevent engorgement. In a successful latch on, the tongue needs to be positioned under the breast with the nipple and areola drawn in. The lips should not be pursed but turned outward and the mouth opened wide. You may need to express a few drops of milk onto your nipple or stroke your baby's cheek or lower lip. Signs of poor latch on by the baby might include sunken cheeks, clicking sounds from broken suction, the tongue not being visible if the lower lip is pulled down, and mom's nipples being creased after nursing.

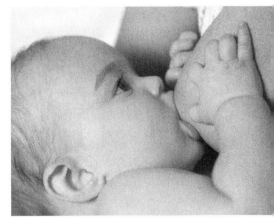

If your baby has trouble latching on, ask your care provider or a lactation consultant for help. He or she may suggest using a breast pump or nipple shields.

"Let-Down" Reflex

Generally, milk doesn't flow from your breast the moment your baby begins to suck. Often it takes a few minutes for the sucking to trigger the let-down reflex, which lets the milk flow. When your baby sucks at your breast and you begin to relax, a surge of the hormone oxytocin in your body prompts your milk glands and ducts to let down the milk.

Many women experience this reflex as a tingling, prickling, almost electrical feeling in their breasts. Besides a baby's suckling, it may be triggered by a crying baby, pumping milk, nipple stimulation, sexual arousal, warm showers, or seemingly nothing at all! This sensation fades as the nursing session progresses, and it frequently disappears altogether after breastfeeding for several months. Whether or not you feel this sensation, you'll know your milk is flowing by listening to your baby's regular, satisfied swallows.

During the first few days or weeks of nursing, the same hormone that makes your milk flow will also make your uterus contract and shrink in size, which can cause mild cramping. These "afterpains" are normal when you nurse, and they'll stop once your uterus has returned to its original size. They can be a useful indicator of a successful latch on and help decrease uterine bleeding. In many cases, afterpains are worse for women who have given birth before.

Supply and Demand

Your milk production is based on supply and demand. The more your baby nurses and the more she empties your breasts, the more milk you'll make. During the first weeks after birth, let her nurse as often as she wants to build up your milk production. If she sucks on an artificial nipple or a pacifier too frequently, she may have trouble latching on to your breast and nursing successfully, which will slow down your milk production. If you're giving your baby supplemental feedings (see page 78), she may be too full to nurse as often as is needed to keep up your milk supply.

If your baby is hungry fairly soon after a nursing session, nurse her again. Soon your breasts will produce enough milk to keep her full for a few hours. You'll know she's getting enough milk by tracking the number of wet and soiled diapers she produces each day, starting a few days after your milk comes in. Dark-yellow urine or dark crystals in baby's urine may be a sign of inadequate hydration. If keeping up your milk supply is an ongoing problem, ask your care provider or a lactation consultant for help. He or she may recommend techniques that will help build up and sustain your milk supply.

Typical soiled diapers when breastfeeding		
Day 1	Meconium stool	1 time
Day 2	Meconium stools	2–3 times
Day 3	Meconium stools may start to transition	4–6 times
Day 4	Meconium stools transitioning to yellow and seedy	6–8 times
Day 5+	Stools should be yellow and seedy	3–4 times

Demand Feeding

Nurse your baby on demand—that is, whenever she's hungry. Don't make a hungry baby wait until a specific time to nurse; doing so may upset both of you. Instead, look for her early hunger cues, like alertness or agitation, opening and closing the mouth, thrusting out the tongue, shaking the head, moving the head toward the breast when held, and sucking on a fist (or on anything!). Nurse your baby frequently, even every hour if necessary.

In the first days to one week of age, a minimum of eight to twelve feedings a day will be necessary. You should wake your newborn at night to feed her if she has slept more than four hours. The more often and longer you nurse, the more milk your breasts produce, which can help prevent the occurrence of potential problems, such as dehydration and the development of jaundice.

Some babies develop a predictable nursing pattern after two or three weeks. For example, they'll nurse once every two to three hours during the day, with longer stretches, every four to five hours, between feedings at night. This pattern is called "cluster feeding." (These are timed from the start of one feeding to the start of the next, not end to start.) Not all babies, however, feed at predictable times, and those who do may change patterns if they're having a growth spurt. A growth spurt often signals a baby to suck more frequently, resulting in more frequent nursing sessions, which encourage your breasts to meet her increasing needs. Typically, babies have growth spurts at two to three weeks, six weeks, three months, and six months. These spurts typically last only a few days. A growth spurt, however, is just one reason why a baby may change her feeding pattern. She may change for no obvious reason.

You will need to wake your baby to nurse if she's losing weight, has jaundice, or is not feeding frequently enough during the day. Once successful feedings are established, your baby should gain 15 to 40 grams a day (one ounce equals 30 grams). Pay attention to your baby's hunger cues, not the clock. The "right" schedule is the one that your baby dictates so she's kept happy and well fed.

Typical weight gain		
Age	Weekly weight gain in ounces	Weekly weight gain in grams
Birth–2 wks.	Regain birth weight	Regain birth weight
2 weeks–6 mos.	5–8	150–240
6–9 mos.	3–5½	90–165
9–12 mos.	2–3	60–90

How Long Should Each Feeding Last?

Let your baby nurse at each breast for as long as she wants, which can vary from five to twenty minutes in order to successfully latch on and transfer enough milk. She'll release the breast when she's full. The length of a feeding often depends on a baby's size and feeding style. Some babies suck vigorously and quickly, and have shorter feedings. Others suck a little, pause, and suck again. Other babies fall asleep at the breast, then wake up and nurse again.

Listen to your baby as she nurses; if she actively sucks and swallows throughout the feeding, she's getting the milk she needs.

Taking Your Baby Off the Breast

Although it's best not to interrupt a nursing session, you may have to remove your baby from the breast for some reason. To do so, gently slip a finger into the corner of your baby's mouth to break the suction.

Which Breast First?

Your baby nurses most vigorously at the first breast you offer, because she's most hungry when she starts. Strong sucking tells your body to produce more milk, so make sure both breasts receive the signal equally by alternating which breast you offer first. (Stick a safety pin on your nursing bra or use a nursing pad to remind you which breast to offer first at the next feeding.) Opinions vary on whether to feed your baby at one or both breasts per individual feeding. There are a few methods you can try. You can nurse at both breasts each feeding, making sure your baby empties the first breast before moving on to the second breast (your baby will receive "hindmilk" from the first breast), then offer the other breast first at the next feeding. You can offer both breasts evenly (but sometimes babies only get "foremilk" and not enough "hindmilk" with this method). Or you can focus on one breast to empty it completely, then offer the other breast at the next feeding (your baby will receive the "hindmilk," but you may not produce as much milk over time).

The "hindmilk" is richer in fat than the thinner "foremilk," which comes out first, and is important for the best growth and development in the baby. Green, frothy stools may be an indicator that your baby is not getting enough "hindmilk." Whatever pattern you settle into over the first few weeks will likely be fine for you if your baby is growing well. Remember to expect your baby to lose 5 to 7 percent of her birth weight in the days after delivery. She is likely to regain her birth weight by one to two weeks of age.

Follow-Up after Hospital Discharge

It is very important that your baby is seen by a health care provider through either a home visit or clinic visit within forty-eight hours after hospital discharge to continue to monitor weight gain, hydration status, feeding progress, and jaundice.

Vitamin Supplements

Over the years, medical opinion has wavered on whether breastfed babies need vitamin supplements. Today, the American Academy of Pediatrics (AAP) recommends that parents give their baby a 400 IU supplement of vitamin D each day beginning soon after birth if she's breastfed exclusively (because she gets only small amounts of vitamin D in breast milk). Vitamin D helps build strong bones (which prevents rickets), strengthens the immune system, and decreases the risk of some chronic diseases such as diabetes. The AAP's recommendation stems from the fact that people produce vitamin D naturally after the skin is exposed to sunshine, but the amount of sunshine newborns are exposed to is unpredictable and inconsistent.

It's also important that nursing moms get adequate amounts of vitamins and minerals in their diets. You can take a prenatal vitamin or a multivitamin-mineral supplement to make sure your breast milk's nutrition is optimal. (For more about your diet, see page 84.)

Supplemental Feedings

Many breastfeeding moms want their babies to be able to take milk from a bottle as well as directly from the breast. During the first few weeks, focus on getting your baby latching on to the breast and sucking effectively. (In individual circumstances where there's a concern of dehydration, hypoglycemia, or an abnormal degree of jaundice, feedings using a supplemental nursing system (SNS), syringe, dropper, or bottle of expressed breast milk or formula may be indicated.) After a few weeks, when she's nursing well, you can introduce her to a bottle (containing expressed milk or formula). Offering a bottle once or twice a week won't interfere with your milk production, and it will teach your baby to feed well from either the breast or bottle. Remember: If your baby has trouble latching on and sucking, don't introduce her to an artificial nipple or pacifier until after successful latch on is established. Sucking on these items may interfere with her ability to nurse successfully. Older infants who have difficulty learning to take a bottle may be able to use a cup instead.

Expressing Milk

Expressing milk lets people other than nursing moms feed a baby breast milk, and it lets working women maintain breastfeeding. (Learn whether your state has laws about continuing to breastfeed in the workplace—it's crucial to know your legal rights if you encounter resistance from your employer. La Leche League has information on individual state laws.) Expressing milk also keeps up mom's milk production and can relieve breast fullness. Some women hand express milk, but breast pumps—electric, battery powered, or manual—offer a great way to express milk more efficiently. They're available to buy or rent. You shouldn't feel any pain or discomfort when expressing milk, and make sure you can remove and clean all pump parts that touch the skin or milk with hot soapy water. If using a breast pump, pump each breast until it's empty to help keep up your milk supply.

Always wash your hands before you pump. Store expressed milk in clean bottles, cups with tight caps, or in special plastic bags (two to four ounces in each). You can place the containers in the freezer or refrigerator. Fresh breast milk can be kept at room temperature for up to four to six hours, and it can be refrigerated for ninety-six hours (four days). Frozen breast milk can be kept in a deep freezer for six months, and it can be kept in the back of an upright freezer for three months. Date all frozen milk, and use the oldest milk first. Never refreeze thawed milk.

Most babies prefer to drink milk warmed to at least room temperature. Never heat breast milk in a microwave; it can cause hot spots and degrades the milk's quality. Microwaved containers also may explode. Instead, warm the container in warm water. Test the temperature of the milk by shaking a few drops onto your wrist.

Breast Pumps

If you're pumping constantly (perhaps because you work full time, your baby is having trouble latching, or you want to build up your milk supply), consider renting a dual-action, hospital-grade pump from a hospital, lactation consultant, or medical supply store. They're the fastest and most efficient type of pump, but also large, very expensive, and generally not available to purchase.

Otherwise, consider buying your own pump. There are three main types:

- Double electric personal-use pumps have powerful motors and rapid suction, and can empty both breasts at the same time. They're the most expensive option (often costing around $300) but typically come with carrying cases and other supplies. These are a good choice for moms who plan to return to work full time and pump often.

- Small electric or battery-operated pumps are lighter and cheaper than automatic models (costing between $50 and $150) but also much slower and usually only capable of emptying one breast at a time. These work best for moms who only need to pump now and then.

- Manual pumps don't require electricity or batteries; moms squeeze a bulb or lever to create suction. This makes manual pumps convenient, but they're also the slowest option and may not completely empty a breast. Moms who rarely pump should choose this option. Manual pumps cost around $30 to $60.

Reverse-Cycle Feeding
If you can't pump milk at work, another option to try is reverse-cycle feeding. This is when you feed your baby more in the evening and at night than during the day (with your baby receiving some daytime supplementation of expressed milk). Your baby will likely sleep more while you're away, and you'll probably want your baby to stay in your room at night, to make feeding easy and increase your bonding time. If you're worried she's not getting enough to eat, check her diapers and weight.

Breast Care

- Wear a nursing bra, even at night, while you're breastfeeding. Buy cotton nursing bras to let your breasts "breathe," and make sure they fit well.
- Air-dry your nipples for fifteen minutes (if possible) after each feeding.
- To help prevent or treat cracked nipples, leave a bit of colostrum or breast milk on your nipples after feedings.
- Shower daily to wash your breasts, but don't use soap. Soap removes natural oils and can lead to cracked nipples. Let them air-dry.
- If your nipples leak, line your bra with thin disposable cotton squares or washable, reusable breast pads to keep your clothes dry. Don't use waterproof liners; they won't let your skin breathe.

Engorgement

When your milk first comes in (usually between two to six days after giving birth), your breasts may feel exceptionally full. This uncomfortable and often painful feeling subsides within a few days, assuming your baby is latching on correctly. (You may also have this feeling later on when your baby goes too long between feedings). In the meantime, nurse frequently to help relieve breast fullness and tenderness. Engorged breasts often make the nipples flat and difficult for your baby to latch on to. Squeeze a few drops of milk onto your nipple to soften it, making it easier for your baby. Wear a supportive bra, which will help push back on the breasts and decrease milk production. You can also take a warm shower or use warm compresses before nursing to help your milk begin dripping from your breasts and make the nipples softer. Once your baby is nursing, gently press on your breasts to encourage milk flow. Switching your baby's position during the feeding may also help milk flow. Let your baby nurse as long as she wants on the first breast. When she stops or falls asleep, offer her the other breast. If she isn't interested, pump or hand-express just enough milk from that breast to relieve the discomfort. If the warm shower or compresses are not of sufficient help, consider applying a cool cloth or ice pack to your breasts after or between feedings to reduce tenderness and swelling. Some care providers suggest taking ibuprofen.

Sore Nipples and Breast Pain

Lots of breastfeeding moms have tender nipples, even those who are nursing their second or third child. Soreness, an abnormality, should be distinguished from tenderness or sensitivity, a normal phenomenon. Soreness and breast pain can have several causes, including injury, engorgement, plugged ducts, infection, dermatitis, and a rare condition called nipple vasoconstriction involving the blood vessels. The soreness can last several days or even weeks. To prevent soreness, make sure your baby learns how to latch on to the nipple appropriately. (See pages 86–87.) Also, wash your nipples with water only and let them air-dry after washing or nursing. If you have a cracked, blistered, or sore nipple (particularly if the soreness gets worse as the baby nurses), try changing your baby's position while nursing to move the pressure to an unaffected area. Bloody nipple discharge may accompany very irritated nipples. A small amount of expressed breast milk on the nipple may help soothe sore nipples. Consult with your care provider or lactation consultant before using creams, oils, or lotions such as those containing lanolin. The temporary use of breast shields and hydrogel pads (available in pharmacies) may also help relieve pain. If nipple pain doesn't improve, have your care provider or a lactation consultant examine your breasts.

Clogged Milk Ducts and Mastitis

When milk doesn't drain completely from the breast, the ducts can become blocked, inflamed, and sore. A clogged duct may be a small, hard, sore lump or a tender spot in your breast.

Several things can cause clogged milk ducts: a tight or ill-fitting bra, shortened or skipped feedings, a bad breast pump, a cold, or stress. Sometimes there may seem to be no reason for them. To help clear a clogged duct, the best remedy is to nurse as often as you can (making sure your baby is in a good position at the breast and that the latch on is correct) and to rest as much as you can. You can also try massaging the sore area or applying warm compresses. Changing your baby's position during a feeding may help, and some affected women claim that positioning the baby so her chin is on the sore spot helps the healing. Some women use herbal remedies like echinacea, lecithin, and vitamin C, and others take ibuprofen sparingly to help relieve the pain and inflammation. Talk with your care provider before taking any herbal remedy or medication.

Left untreated, a clogged duct can turn into a bacterial breast infection called mastitis. An infected breast becomes red and tender, and the infection can cause fever, aches, and nausea. Mastitis won't harm your baby. To treat it, continue nursing your baby, because removing the milk helps clear up the infection. If nursing is extremely painful, offer only the uninfected breast. Also, contact your care provider; he or she will likely prescribe antibiotics to destroy the infection and may prescribe acidophilus to prevent you from getting a yeast infection. A breast abscess, a very localized and more serious infection, can rarely develop and requires immediate medical attention.

Yeast Infection (Candida)

A yeast infection of the breast often occurs following an antibiotic treatment or when you have a vaginal yeast infection. It can also occur when your baby has a yeast diaper rash or thrush (a yeast infection of the mouth). A yeast infection may possibly make your nipples pinker and more irritated, and it can make them very painful with tingling and burning during and between feedings. Sometimes the affected nipple can become shiny or flaky. If either you or your baby has a yeast infection—with or without visible symptoms—you'll both need treatment. Talk with your care provider for treatment suggestions, which may include an antifungal cream, oral medication, or liquid medication to apply to your nipples. A skin culture or culture from breast milk can help confirm a yeast infection. (See page 209 for more information about thrush.)

Hiccups

Your baby may get the hiccups while nursing; this is normal. She can continue feeding, and the hiccups will stop on their own.

Biting

Your baby may bite your nipples as she nurses. This is more likely if she is orally defensive (will not allow anything to approach her mouth), has a recessed jaw, or has tongue-tie. When your baby gets teeth, around three to twelve months, it can hurt! (Some babies are born with teeth, called natal teeth, and though this is uncommon the teeth may need to be smoothed or removed.) Know that she's not being malicious, nor does her biting suggest she wants to be weaned. Rather, it's likely that her new teeth—or teeth that have yet to break through—are bothering her gums, and biting on anything makes them feel better.

This doesn't mean you should ignore it when your baby bites you. Biting typically occurs at the end of a feeding, when she's full and is simply playing. As soon as you feel a bite, gently but firmly say no and remove her from the breast. Also offer teething rings or toys as a more suitable biting object. Using these approaches consistently should teach her not to bite on your breast.

Tongue-Tie (Ankyloglossia)

Some babies have a piece of tissue between the bottom of the tongue and the floor of the mouth that's shorter and tauter than usual and may keep them from moving their tongue properly. This usually does not interfere with correct latch on, but in some cases it helps to have the tissue cut (a procedure called a frenotomy) to facilitate successful latch on and suckling. Your care provider or lactation consultant should be able to help diagnose this problem.

Premature Babies, Ill Babies, and Multiple Babies

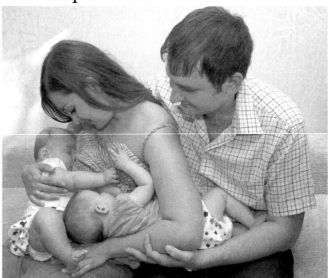

Many premature or ill babies can breast-feed. In fact, breast milk provides the best nutrition to help growth, and because it contains antibodies from mom, it can help prevent diseases (especially important for premature babies, who have a harder time fighting off infections). The swallowing mechanisms of premature babies are less mature, however, and may make breastfeeding difficult. If you can't breastfeed your baby, you should express milk—preferably at least eight times a day—and give the milk to your baby through a feeding tube, syringe, cup, or bottle. Moms of multiples will have more than one mouth to feed, and many learn to nurse two babies simultaneously, one at each breast. It's important for nursing moms of multiples to have the support of lactation consultants and breastfeeding organizations like La Leche League to ensure that all of their babies are getting the nutrition they need.

Support for Nursing Moms

Although breastfeeding your baby is natural, it still requires commitment and practice. Problems, like engorgement and infection, discourage some women. Working moms may feel uncomfortable expressing milk on the job or find it too time consuming. Some feel nursing chains them to their babies, that they can't go anywhere because they must be ready for the next feeding.

Nursing moms need emotional support as well as practical information. Breastfeeding organizations, like La Leche League (LLL), are designed to provide you with support and encouragement. Most communities have a local LLL chapter that holds regular meetings. Many communities also have lactation consultants who can help establish and support breastfeeding. More and more health care facilities have breastfeeding specialists on staff. Take advantage of the professional breastfeeding support you may have in your area.

Milk Banks

If you can't provide your baby with breast milk, you may want to use donor milk from a milk bank. Milk banks collect, screen, process, and distribute milk to those who need it, particularly babies who are premature or ill. There are currently seventeen banks in the United States and three in Canada that follow the safety guidelines of the Human Milk Banking Association of North America (HMBANA). These banks carefully screen and pasteurize the donated milk before sending it out. (Giving your baby milk that hasn't been screened isn't safe. For this reason, buying milk over the Internet from other sources is not recommended). For more information, see their website, http://www.hmbana.org/.

What Nursing Moms Need

Rest

Getting enough rest is essential to good milk production, especially during the first weeks of breastfeeding. Your body is still recovering from giving birth, and inadequate rest may make you feel more stress, which often interferes with milk production. Try to sleep when your baby naps, and ignore all those tasks you'd like to get done. They'll get done eventually, but now is the time to focus on you and your baby.

Relaxation

Relax as much as you can, especially just before you nurse your baby. Emotional and physical tension (including stress, anxiety, and illness) can interfere with your let-down reflex and milk supply, which can keep your baby from getting the milk she needs. Try settling into a comfortable chair and turning on some soothing music before a feeding.

Liquids

Nursing mothers need to drink plenty of liquids (six to eight glasses a day). Get into the habit of drinking a glass of water or another liquid before or with each feeding. You may be more thirsty while nursing. Don't force yourself to drink, though. Just drink enough to quench your thirst. Pale-yellow urine is a good sign you're drinking enough.

Medications

Many medications are safe to take while breastfeeding. But before taking any medication—prescribed or over the counter—talk first with your care provider or lactation consultant. Moms who have insulin resistance and take combined estrogen/progestin contraceptives may experience breastfeeding problems.

Diet

When breastfeeding, your body will use nutrients to make breast milk first, then it'll nourish itself. Unless you're extremely malnourished, whatever you eat will usually provide good-quality breast milk; however, your diet can affect *how much* milk you produce and your overall health. A nursing mom needs to increase her caloric intake over her baseline by 25 percent (so if you usually eat two thousand calories a day, you'll need to add five hundred calories), and her diet, in addition to being well rounded, should include about 65 grams of protein and plenty of calcium as well as some vitamins and trace minerals. (If you're worried about your weight, remember that breastfeeding burns five hundred calories a day, on average.) A guideline for your diet follows. (For a personalized daily food plan, see http://www.choosemyplate.gov.)

A few things to keep in mind:

- Teen mothers who nurse will need more dairy and protein. Moms of multiples may need to add one thousand calories to this daily diet. If you're a teen or a mom of multiples, talk with your care provider or a nutritionist about your nutritional needs for breastfeeding.
- If there is a family history of food allergies, you may need to be more restrictive in your diet. Research is actively continuing in this area. (See page 182 for more on food allergies.)

- Some foods you eat may cause problems for your nursing baby.
  - Try limiting foods that cause gas (like cabbage, broccoli, garlic, and onions) if you notice she's fussy when you eat these foods.
  - Caffeine can also make your baby fussy. Many moms, however, are able to consume caffeine in moderate amounts (a serving or two) without problems.
  - Some babies are allergic to the protein in cow's milk. If you think your baby is allergic, don't eat or drink anything containing cow's milk for two weeks to see if the symptoms (eczema or skin rash, abdominal pain or cramps, vomiting, or diarrhea) disappear.
- It's best if you don't regularly consume large amounts of alcohol or smoke cigarettes at any time in your life—but especially not while breastfeeding. (Contrary to earlier beliefs, beer consumption has not been shown to increase milk supply.) Alcohol in your bloodstream crosses over into your milk and may change the taste of the milk. Large amounts of alcohol can harm your nursing baby as well as impair your caretaking abilities. But drinking alcohol *in moderation* (an occasional single drink) is possible if you're careful. A single drink is defined as twelve ounces of beer, four ounces of wine, or one ounce of hard liquor. Consider feeding your baby before having a drink, to give yourself time for the alcohol to leave your system before you nurse her again. You should allow at least two hours after one drink before your next breastfeeding. If you're exposed to cigarette smoke while nursing, so is your baby. If you just can't quit smoking, it's better to smoke and breastfeed than to smoke and not breastfeed, and you should smoke right after you nurse, and well away from your baby. (Make sure if anyone else smokes, he or she does so well away from you and your baby.) For more information, talk with your care provider about using alcohol and tobacco while breastfeeding.
- Fish intake has the potential to contribute healthy omega-3 fatty acids to your baby. Fish also contain mercury, however, which crosses into the baby through breast milk. Current guidelines suggest fish intake should be eight to twelve ounces per week, which is equal to two average servings. The types of fish and shellfish recommended are those with the lowest concentrations of mercury, such as shrimp, canned light tuna, salmon, pollack, and catfish. Albacore tuna should be limited to six ounces per week. If you eat locally caught fish, check the advisories in your specific area for guidelines.

Food Groups	Daily Servings	Sources
Dairy	3 cups	Cheese, custard, milk, pudding, yogurt
Protein	6½ oz.	Fish, dried beans, lean beef or pork, lentils, poultry, eggs (Caution: The protein in nuts and nut butter can appear in breast milk. If you have a family history of severe allergies or asthma, discuss this with your baby's care provider.)
Fruits and Vegetables	5½ cups	Dark-green leafy vegetables, orange and red vegetables, variety of fruits including kiwi fruit, avocados, oranges
Grains	9 oz.	Bread, bulgur, cereals, pancakes, pasta, rice (preferably whole grain)
Sweets and Fats	Moderate amounts	Chips, cookies, candy

Nursing Positions

For all nursing positions, make sure your infant's face is facing your body so her mouth is opposite your nipple with her neck slightly extended and her head, shoulders, and hips in alignment.

Cradle Hold, Cross Cradle Hold Step-by-Step

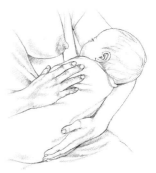

Step 1: Sit with your baby in a comfortable chair. You may find using a footstool helpful, as well as pillows to help support your baby. (There are specially designed pillows to help bring your baby up to the level of the breast.) Lay the side of your baby's head in the crook of your arm. Support her body with your arm, and support her bottom with your hand. You and your baby should be belly to belly. Wrap her bottom arm around your side so it's not wedged between the two of you.

Another way to hold your baby is to rest her head in your hand and support her body with your arm, letting her bottom rest in the crook of your arm. This is called the alternate or cross cradle hold, and some nursing moms find it an easier position to master than the regular cradle hold.

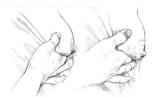

Step 2: Make a "breast sandwich" with your other hand by placing the fingers on one side of your breast and the thumb on the other side, at least two inches away from the areola.

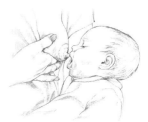

Step 3: Pull your baby close to you. Tickle her upper lip with your nipple until her mouth opens wide.

Step 4: Center your nipple in front of your baby's nose so she'll latch on to it. If you discover the nipple is not properly centered after your baby has latched on, you can try changing its position by pressing your thumb or fingers into the breast. But this method can move the nipple into an incorrect position, usually leading to a sore nipple. If the nipple isn't centered when your baby first latches on, it's best to just take her off the breast (gently stick a finger in the corner of her mouth to break the suction) and try again.

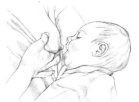

Step 5: When your baby has latched on properly, her bottom lip will flange out around the breast. If it's curled inward over her lower gum, pull gently on her chin until her lip flanges outward. Other signs of a good latch include your baby's cheek against your breast, audible swallowing, and overall comfort for you and your baby throughout the feeding.

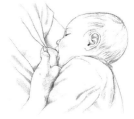

Side-Lying Step-by-Step

(You may prefer this method if you've undergone a cesarean section, because it'll keep your baby off your belly.)

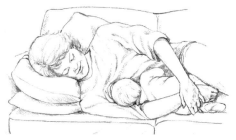

Step 1: Lie on your side on a bed or roomy couch with pillows around your head and shoulders.

Step 2: Curve your body slightly so your baby can fit comfortably next to you.

Step 3: Lay your baby on her side, slightly raising and supporting her head in the crook of your arm. Wrap your forearm around her and draw her feet close to you so she's angled into your body. This position will help keep her nose free to breathe while she's nursing.

Step 4: Be sure you're supported entirely by the furniture and pillows, not by your back muscles or elbow. Then follow steps 2 through 5 for the Cradle Hold.

> *Note:* It's important that your baby does not sleep with your breast in her mouth. Pooled milk (with its milk sugar) can cause dental decay in erupting teeth. Babies who feed lying down also have a greater chance of getting ear infections.

Football Hold (Clutch) Step-by-Step

(You may prefer this method if you've undergone a cesarean section, because it'll keep your baby off your belly. It also can be preferable for premature babies, and multiples.)

Step 1: Use a comfortable, well-padded chair or rocker. You may want to place a pillow behind your back for support or under your baby so she's in a more convenient position to nurse.

Step 2: Avoid leaning forward while nursing. You'll end up with a backache.

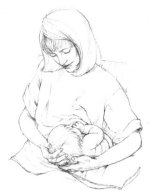

Step 3: Support your baby in the football position (see page 24), turning her toward you at your side.

Step 4: Support your baby's head so it's higher than her stomach. This position lets her better burp up any swallowed air. Then follow steps 2 through 5 for the Cradle Hold.

> *Note:* For further information on burping, see page 97.

Weaning from the Breast

When?

There's no one specific time when your baby should be weaned, but it's recommended that babies breastfeed for at least the first one to two years of life.

During the first year, your baby may suddenly stop breastfeeding. At this age, her refusal usually doesn't suggest she's ready to be weaned. More likely, she's on a "nursing strike." A change in the nursing routine or schedule, a change in your stress level, or even a change in the deodorant or soap you use may make your baby refuse to nurse. If your baby is six months or older, general distraction may be the reason for her loss of interest in nursing. With your patience and persistence, she should resume nursing. Talk with your care provider or a lactation consultant for help getting your baby back on the breast.

Babies who self-wean usually do so gradually over a period of several weeks or months. Self-weaning is often the least traumatic and problem-free way of weaning. If, however, you decide to wean your baby, she may need extra attention, especially if you've been nursing for a long time. Try to give her all the cuddling and care you can.

> In rare instances, babies are weaned during the first year if their mothers have a serious medical condition that requires drugs incompatible with breastfeeding. If you're in this situation, refer to the AAP, WHO, and CDC websites for lists of incompatible medication, and get a second opinion from another care provider before starting the medication. Depending on the age of your baby and how often she nurses, certain drugs might not harm her.

How?

How you wean may be more important than *when* you wean. When it's time, do it gradually, gently, and with plenty of love and patience.

- Be as flexible as you can. Don't set strict goals or rigid schedules.

- Avoid sudden weaning for two reasons. It can dramatically decrease your hormonal flow, which could trigger depression—and the loss of the nursing bond with your child may add to the depression. Sudden weaning can also traumatize your baby, who's learned to find comfort and solace, as well as nourishment, from nursing. Engorgement will likely result as well.

- Gradually cut back one feeding at a time every two to three days. Also shorten the time of the other feedings and increase the time between them as well. The lunchtime or midday feeding is usually the first one to go. Many babies cling longest to the bedtime or first morning feeding. Offer your baby expressed breast milk, formula, or water from a cup or a bottle in addition to food (if she's started eating solids). If you wean to a bottle, choose a nipple with a slow flow. Every two to three days, substitute another bottle or cup feeding for the breastfeeding. Many babies can be weaned entirely in one to two weeks.

- If you're weaning from breast milk to formula or cow's milk, and your baby doesn't like the taste, try a mixture of half breast milk and half formula or cow's milk.
- If your baby weans early, she may miss sucking, especially at bedtime. Offer her a cup, pacifier, or bottle. (Don't offer a bottle to your baby in bed.)
- Except for very young infants, most babies often can be weaned directly to a cup. A weighted two-handled cup with a valveless spout works especially well for an inexperienced drinker.
- If you wean your baby gradually, you'll probably avoid engorged breasts. (See page 80.) If your breasts become uncomfortably full after a missed feeding, express some milk—but just until you're fairly comfortable again. (See pages 78–79.) Don't express too much, or you'll stimulate more milk production. Try to avoid pumping if possible.
- If your baby is weaning well and suddenly suffers from teething or a cold, she'll probably want to nurse. Don't deny her this comfort while she's miserable. When she starts to feel better, you can resume weaning.

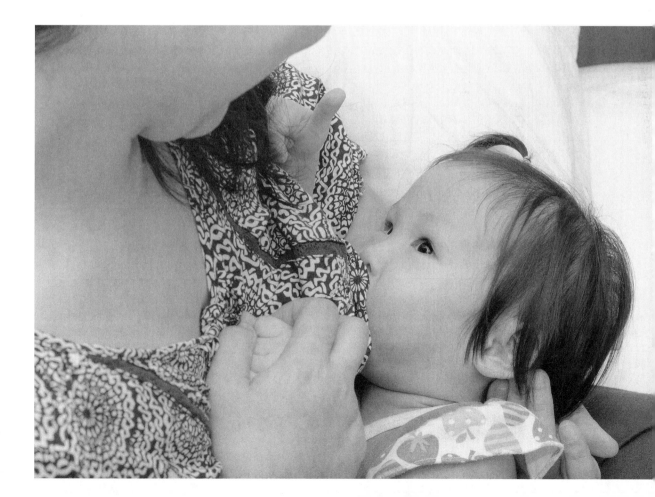

Formula-Feeding Basics

This section focuses on how to feed your baby formula, but you can also follow the steps on pages 78-79 to learn how to feed expressed breast milk to your baby. In the United States, the Food and Drug Administration (FDA) regulates and monitors all commercial infant formulas. It is not safe to give your baby homemade formulas or cow or other animal milk (in the first year) as a source of nutrition.

Kinds of Formula

Formula comes in several different forms and many different compositions. Formula companies are constantly changing and updating their products, usually striving to make them closer in constitution to breast milk. Formulas vary slightly among brands, but the cost of brands can vary more significantly. Most companies add vitamins to their formula, making additional vitamin supplements unnecessary. (It is recommended, however, to give additional vitamin D to formula-fed babies early on, before they are up to an intake of thirty-two ounces a day.) The American Academy of Pediatrics (AAP) recommends iron-fortified formula for all formula-fed babies for the first year to promote normal mental and physical development. Some parents worry that lots of iron will make their baby constipated. Actually, iron can cause either diarrhea or constipation, but it usually causes neither. If constipation becomes a problem, you can treat it while still giving your baby iron-fortified formula. (See page 166.) Most babies do well on the first formula they consume, and switching formulas should not be done without input from a care provider. Discuss with your baby's care provider which formula he or she recommends for your baby.

There are three main kinds of commercially prepared formulas:

- *Milk-based* formula is made with cow's milk that has been modified to be more like breast milk and fortified with vitamins, minerals, carbohydrates, and non–milk fats. About 80 percent of formula sold is milk based. Some milk-based formulas are "lactose-free," but these generally aren't needed except in some postdiarrhea circumstances. When babies have milk intolerance, the problem is usually the protein, not the sugar (lactose), in milk.

- *Soy-based* formula is made from soybeans (this is vegetable, not animal, based) and is also fortified with vitamins, minerals, carbohydrates, and fats. It's usually consumed by babies who are allergic to the protein in cow's milk, or are lactose intolerant. (It should be noted, however, that as many as 50 percent of babies who have milk-protein allergy also have soy-protein allergy.) Once again, lactose-free formulas are generally not needed by babies except occasionally in postdiarrhea circumstances.

- *Hydrolyzed* formula is cow's milk–based but with the proteins broken down to various degrees to make them more digestible. Sometimes these are referred to as predigested formulas. Types may be listed as gentle, sensitive, or hypoallergenic. This formula is helpful for babies with severe protein sensitivity or allergy but is about twice as expensive as regular cow's milk or soy formula.

- Formulas may list other features, including added lipids or fatty acids such as docosa-hexaenoic acid (DHA) and arachidonic acid (ARA), prebiotics (natural food substances that promote a healthy intestinal lining) and probiotics ("friendly" bacteria), or organic ingredients. These additions help formula imitate breast milk even more and are generally felt to be advantageous. Other options on the market are organic and non-GMO formulas. Generics are an acceptable and less expensive option.

Infant formulas come packaged three ways:
- *Ready-to-feed* formula is premixed and ready to pour into a clean bottle. This is the most expensive formula but also the most convenient.
- *Powdered* formula must be mixed with water. The standard recipe is one scoop of formula per two ounces of water. You can prepare one bottle of formula at a time.
- *Concentrated liquid* formula must be diluted with water before it's poured into a bottle. The standard recipe is equal parts water to formula.

If you use powdered or concentrated liquid formulas, dilute with fluoride-free water—the formula already provides enough fluoride for your baby in her first year. If you are using well water, have the water tested to make sure it is safe for your baby.

Storing Formula

- Once you've opened a container of concentrated or ready-to-use formula and prepared bottles, cover and store the remaining formula in the refrigerator for up to forty-eight hours. After that time, throw it out.
- Once you've opened a can of powdered formula, cover the can and store it in a cool, dry place. The label will tell you how long you can use the formula.
- After you've prepared a bottle of formula, either use it immediately or refrigerate it. You can safely use prepared formula for twenty-four to forty-eight hours after it's been refrigerated.
- If you'll be away from your home for more than two hours, bring the supplies to pre-pare formula with you instead of preparing at home, to keep freshness longer.
- You can leave a prepared bottle at room temperature for up to two hours before bac-teria starts to grow in the formula (a half hour in very warm weather). After an hour, throw out the formula if your baby has eaten some of it. (Bacteria from her mouth will grow in the formula.) If she hasn't eaten any of it, you can safely refrigerate the bottle and use it up to forty-eight hours later.

Preparing Formula

Tips

- With common sense and good hygiene, there's no need to sterilize any of the feeding equipment or the water you use. Clean the equipment regularly, and carefully wash your hands in hot soapy water before you prepare the formula.

- Prepare the formula exactly as your baby's care provider prescribes or as the formula manufacturer recommends. Formula that's too concentrated or too diluted can make your baby sick.
- Follow the steps on page 94 to prepare powdered or concentrated formula. A ready-to-use formula needs no preparation; simply pour it into a clean bottle.

Equipment

There are a number of bottle and nipple styles to choose from. Your baby may prefer a particular nipple, and you may find that some bottle systems are more convenient for you than others. The following list suggests how many bottles and nipples you'll need; it also outlines the advantages of various nipple and bottle features. You may want to buy a sample of each style in the beginning, then let your baby and your budget help you decide which to stock up on.

Bottles, 8–10 (plus 8–10 caps or covers and screw-on rings)	
Feature	Description
Material	Glass bottles are durable, easy to clean, and don't contain harmful chemicals, but they're heavier than plastic bottles and can shatter if dropped or thrown.
	Plastic bottles are light and won't shatter, but they might not last as long as glass bottles.
	Stainless steel bottles are light and won't shatter, are easy to clean and very durable.
Shape	Straight bottles are cheap and easy to clean.
	Angled bottles have a forty-five-degree bend that keeps the nipple filled with liquid to reduce baby's air intake and makes it easier to hold a baby upright, which prevents liquid from washing into baby's middle ear (a cause of ear infections).
Usage	Reusable bottles are economical and environmentally sound because they can be used throughout your baby's bottle-feeding stage and create no waste. They also allow accurate measurement of the bottle's contents.
	Disposable bottles (with liners) require less cleaning because the milk is drunk from a pre-sterilized plastic liner, which is thrown away at the end of the feeding. This bottle type may minimize baby's air swallowing (and thus prevent gassiness) because you can squeeze air out of the liner before feeding; also, the liner collapses as baby feeds, which prevents additional air bubbles from entering.
Size	Four-ounce bottles are practical for newborns, who may drink only a small amount at each feeding. They're also handy for storing expressed breast milk.
	Eight- or nine-ounce bottles are most practical for older babies with bigger appetites, but they can be used for a baby of any age and are therefore more versatile and long lasting.
Other features	Bubble-free bottles are ideal for gassy babies (if you'd rather not use disposable bottles). They let air in through the bottom of the bottle, which prevents it from mixing with the milk and being swallowed. Because both ends screw off, cleaning is easy.
	Chambered bottles are great for traveling with a formula-fed baby. They have separate compartments for premeasured powdered formula and water. At feeding time, you twist the top and the formula mixes with the water.
	Hands-free bottle systems have been redesigned to be safer than in past years. Because the use of a hands-free bottle system gets in the way of the important bonding that takes place during feeding, try to minimize its use (although it may be particularly helpful for young multiples). Never leave a baby unattended while using a hands-free bottle system.

Nipples	
Feature	**Description**
Material	Latex nipples are softer and more flexible than silicone nipples.
	Silicone nipples are firmer and hold their shape longer than latex ones. They're less porous than latex and thus less prone to bacteria. They typically last three to four times longer than latex. They're also heat resistant and can withstand dishwashers.
Shape	Bell-shaped nipples are inexpensive and widely available.
	Flat-topped nipples mimic the shape of a mother's nipple.
	Orthodontic nipples are elongated, flat on one side, and indented in the center to encourage the tonguing action of breastfeeding. They may help reduce tongue thrusting and bite problems caused by standard nipples.
Flow	Nipples come with holes in varying numbers and sizes for varying flow speed. Here's a quick guide to choosing the right flow: Always use "newborn" or "stage 1" nipples for a breastfed baby of any age. The following guidelines apply to exclusively bottle-fed babies. For a newborn, the nipple size is right if the milk drips steadily when you turn the bottle upside down. For older babies, if your baby is sucking hard, fussing, then sucking hard again, you probably need a faster-flow nipple. If your baby is sputtering and gulping, you may need a slower-flow nipple.

Other Basic Equipment

- Bottle brush
- Nipple brush
- Measuring pitcher in ounces (or milliliters), preferably one with a cover
- Funnel
- Large, long-handled spoon

Care of Equipment

- Thoroughly rinse the formula from each bottle immediately after it's used.
- Wash each bottle, ring, and nipple separately in hot soapy water, using the nipple and bottle brushes. Carefully squeeze water through the nipples to remove all residue. You can also wash everything in the dishwasher.
- Rinse everything in clean hot water and let air-dry.

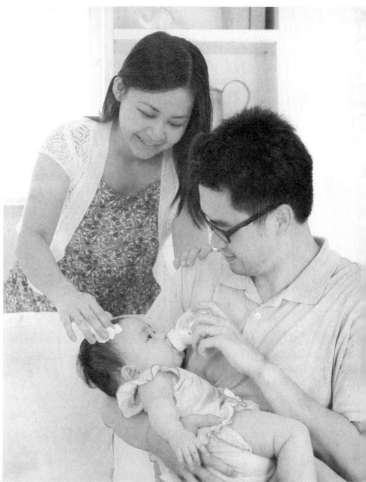

Preparing Formula Step-by-Step

Step 1: Wash your hands thoroughly with hot soapy water. If you're opening a can of concentrated formula, clean the top of the can.

Step 2: Prepare the formula exactly as recommended to keep your baby from getting sick. Pour the formula into clean bottles. Using a funnel makes the job easier.

Step 3: Put the nipples, rings, and caps on the bottles. Store the bottles in the refrigerator. (See page 91 to learn how to store formula safely.)

How Much?

- Begin by offering your baby about one-half to one and a half ounces (15 to 45 milliliters) at each feeding for the first few days. Work up to two to three ounces (60 to 90 milliliters) per feeding from one to three weeks. Expect her to eat about every three to four hours on average during the first weeks. As soon as she starts emptying the bottle at two or three feedings each day, start adding half an ounce (15 milliliters) of formula to each bottle. Expect her to work up to twelve to twenty-four ounces a day. Eventually, she'll drink eight ounces (240 millimeters) a feeding. No more than thirty-two ounces of formula should be given in twenty-four hours. You can follow these rough guidelines for the first year, but let your baby decide how much food she wants.
- Don't worry if your baby doesn't drink much formula at a feeding. Just as your appetite fluctuates, so does hers. If she's happy and thriving, it's usually okay if she doesn't drink much once in a while.
- Sometimes a baby will stop sucking during a feeding. Be patient; she's probably just resting. When she's ready, she'll start again. Don't force a bottle if it's clear she doesn't want any more, and don't pressure her to finish a bottle if she clearly isn't interested.

Age	Amount each day
Birth to 1 mo.	12–24 oz. (530–710 ml)
1 to 2 mos.	22–26 oz. (650–770 ml)
2–3 mos.	24–26 oz. (710–770 ml)
3–4 mos.	24–28 oz. (710–830 ml)

Age	Amount each day
4–5 mos.	24–30 oz. (710–890 ml)
5–6 mos.	24–32 oz. (710–950 ml)
6 mos. to 1 yr.	24–32 oz. (710–950 ml)

Demand Feeding

- Let your baby's hunger determine when she'll be fed. Feeding her whenever she seems hungry won't spoil her. (See hunger cues on page 76.) Bottle-fed babies usually feed every three to four hours. They eventually need fewer feedings at night.
- You usually don't need to wake your baby at night for a feeding after one to two months. If she's hungry, she'll wake herself.

Giving the Bottle to Your Baby

Tips

- Most babies prefer their formula or milk slightly warm, although some like it cooler. If you're using tap water to make a bottle, make sure it does not contain a significant amount of lead (more than 15 parts per billion or ppb); call the EPA's Safe Drinking Water Hotline at 800-426-4791 for more information. If there is lead in your water, it's better to use cold water than warm water. To warm a cold bottle, set it in a pan of warm water. Do not warm the bottle in the microwave. Using a microwave can cause hot spots that can scald the baby's mouth, and it can make the bottle break. Make sure the liquid isn't too hot by dripping a bit on the inside of your wrist (where your skin is more sensitive to temperature than your hands).

- Check the flow of milk from the nipple. The milk should drip out steadily—initially about one drop per second. If it drips too slowly, your baby will tire of sucking before she's full and will probably swallow a lot of air instead. If the milk comes out too quickly, your baby will get full before she's sucked as much as she needs to. Plus, she may try to slow the flow by thrusting her tongue against the nipple, which can affect the development of her teeth. Throw away the nipple if the milk flows too quickly.

- Avoid propping a bottle or teaching your young baby to hold it herself before she learns to do it naturally. If left alone with a bottle, a baby could choke on the liquid.

- Be attentive and remember that every baby needs the cuddling and love that comes while feeding.

- Avoid putting your baby to bed with a bottle. A baby who feeds lying down has a greater chance of getting an ear infection. Plus, falling asleep with a bottle in her mouth can lead to severe tooth decay, even if she hasn't yet cut her teeth.

Step-by-Step

Step 1: Hold your baby on your lap, nestled in the crook of your arm. Gently touch her nearest cheek with the nipple to trigger her rooting reflex (see page 21). She'll turn toward you with an open mouth, searching for the nipple.

Step 2: Hold your baby with her head and upper body raised at a slight angle. She'll more easily swallow the formula or milk in this position than if she's lying on her back.

Step 3: Keep the neck of the bottle constantly filled with liquid by gradually lifting the bottom of the bottle as you feed your baby. She'll swallow more liquid and less air. When your baby's finished, burp her. (See page 97 for instructions.)

Weaning from the Bottle

When?

There's no one specific time when your baby should be weaned, but weaning can be easier when she's old enough to drink from a cup by herself (as early as five or six months old). Many bottle-fed babies who can drink from a cup are weaned completely by their first birthdays. Weaning to a cup earlier rather than later can prevent the bottle from becoming a security object. Plus, drinking from a cup improves hand-to-mouth coordination.

Signs that your baby may be ready to wean include: looking around while sucking on the bottle, mouthing the nipple instead of sucking on it, and putting down the bottle before she's finished it.

How?

How you wean may be more important than *when* you wean. When it's time, do it gradually, gently, and with plenty of love and patience.

- Occasionally offer your baby formula or water in a cup. A weighted two-handled cup with a valveless spout works especially well for an inexperienced drinker.
- If your baby loves her bottle and refuses to drink from a cup, continue offering the cup to her. When she eventually starts taking a sip or two, don't force her to drink more. She'll do so when she's ready.
- Gradually cut back one bottle feeding at a time. The lunchtime feeding is usually the first to go. Many babies cling longest to the bedtime or first morning feeding.
- If your baby is weaning well and suddenly suffers from teething or a cold, she'll probably want a bottle. Don't deny her this comfort while she's miserable. When she starts to feel better, you can resume weaning.

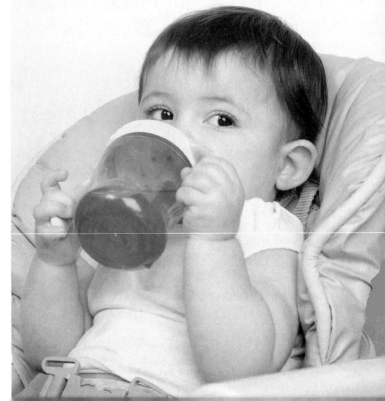

Burping and Spitting Up

Tips

- Bottle-fed babies tend to swallow air as they feed, making them uncomfortable until they burp. (Breastfed babies might swallow air, too, if their mouths don't create a tight seal as they nurse or if they nurse while flat on their backs.)

- Unless your baby is very fussy, it's usually enough to burp her once during a feeding and once after. It may be helpful to burp a bottle-fed baby after she's eaten two or three ounces (or at least every three to five minutes) to help reduce the amount of any swallowed air.

- Don't interrupt your baby's feeding to burp her. Take advantage of her pauses in sucking and burp her then. If nursing, burp her before you offer your second breast.

- If your baby doesn't burp within a few minutes, resume feeding her and try again later if she's fussy.

- Before you burp your baby, drape a cloth diaper or towel over your shoulder or knees to catch any spit-up.

- Spitting up some formula or milk with a burp is normal. It happens when the stomach muscles gently dispel some formula or milk. (Vomiting, as a comparison, is when the stomach muscles vigorously contract and dispel most of the formula or milk.) Swallowing too much air or eating too much at a feeding often results in spit-up, especially for bottle-fed babies. Sometimes, though, it's due to relaxation of the muscles that control the passage between the stomach and the esophagus (or *reflux*—see pages 184–85 for more information). Your baby will spit up less often as she grows.

- Don't bounce or jiggle your baby after a feeding. Doing so may make her spit up.

- To help prevent spit-up, keep your baby upright for a half hour after feeding.

- If your baby spits up a lot of formula or milk, hold her in a more upright position when you feed her so any swallowed air isn't trapped below the formula or milk in her stomach.

Burping Methods

Option 1: Hold your baby with her head over your shoulder. Gently rub or pat her back until she burps.

Option 2: Set your baby upright and leaning slightly forward on your lap. Support her head and body. Gently rub or pat her back until she burps.

Option 3: Lay your baby facedown across your lap or on a mattress. Turn her head to one side and support it with your hand or arm. Gently rub or pat her back until she burps.

Introducing Solid (Complementary) Foods

When your baby is six months old, she may be ready to start eating solids. Unlike when breast milk or formula was all your baby ate, you'll now be concerned that she's eating a well-balanced diet. Once she starts deciding what she will or won't eat, you realize that you don't have total control over her diet. (*You* may think she needs to eat strained peas, but *she* may think otherwise.) Your baby may be an easygoing eater, a vigorous masher, an energetic thrower, or a combination of all types, depending on the time of day, her mood, or who knows what! Do not introduce solids by adding them into a bottle unless specifically advised by your health care provider.

When?

For your baby's health, the American Academy of Pediatrics (AAP) recommends waiting to introduce solids to her until she's six months old. At that age, her body may be ready for the additional calories and nutrients that solid foods offer. When your baby's ready to try solid foods, her usual intake of breast milk or formula may no longer satisfy her. Make sure, however, that her demand for more feedings isn't due to a growth spurt. (Growth spurts usually occur at two to three weeks, six weeks, three months, and six months—but the demand for more food lasts only two or three days for each spurt.) Your baby may also give you some of the following cues to show she's ready to eat solid foods:

• She sits well with minimal support.

• She can support and control her head well; watch for this when she's sitting in a high chair, feeding seat, or infant seat.

• When lying facedown, she can push up with straight elbows.

• She tries to take food off your plate or grab your fork.

• She turns her head away when she's done drinking or eating.

• She has lost the tongue thrust (extrusion) reflex. (See page 21.)

• She opens her mouth when she sees the food-laden spoon approaching.

• She is big enough, as indicated by having doubled her birth weight.

Why Wait?

Before they're six months old, most babies' digestive systems aren't developed enough to process solids effectively and safely. Many babies can't control their tongue and mouth muscles well enough to swallow solid foods safely. This could lead to your baby inhaling liquid or food into her lungs (called aspiration).

Plus, if you're nursing your baby, breast milk is designed to provide all the nutrition she needs until she's ready to eat solid foods. Feeding her solids too soon only fills her with nutritionally inferior foods.

Here are a few more reasons to delay introducing solids to your baby:

- Delaying the introduction of solid foods may help avoid food allergies and allergic conditions like eczema and asthma. If your baby's digestive tract isn't mature enough, the large proteins found in solid foods can sometimes get through the lining of her intestinal wall. If this happens, her immune system kicks in and produces antibodies, resulting in an allergic reaction.
- Introducing solid foods too early may contribute to obesity later on. A 2011 study by the AAP found that, among formula-fed infants, introducing solid foods before age four months was related to a higher risk of obesity.
- Contrary to popular belief, it's never been clearly demonstrated that mixing cereal in a baby's bedtime bottle will help her sleep through the night. In fact, the practice may do your baby more harm than good.

How to Introduce Solids

Keep in mind the following suggestions when your baby is ready to try a solid food:

- Introduce solid foods while your baby is still getting most of her nourishment from breast milk or formula. Offer solids at any time of the day you prefer and either before or after she's nursed or had a bottle. Solids should supplement, not replace, breast milk or formula.
- Offer solids on a small spoon, not in a bottle, unless specifically instructed to do so for gastroesophageal reflux disease. Also, do not introduce pureed food by letting your baby suck it out of a pouch; these pouches are convenient for travel but should not be used during the introduction period.
- Offer your baby solids when she's active and calm.
- Don't force your baby to eat solids. She'll eat when her body needs them. Introducing solid foods should be an enjoyable, stress-free activity.
- Respect your baby's preferences. Even at six months old, she'll have likes and dislikes. Still, it can take ten to fifteen tries (maybe even more) for a baby to accept a new food. Don't give up on a food just because your baby spits it out for the first, fifth, or twelfth time!
- At first, introduce solids one at a time. Wait at least two to four days after each new food to make sure it doesn't cause an allergic reaction. If your family has a history of allergies, wait a full week before offering the food again. Avoid stews, soups, or multi-grain cereals; if any of these causes an allergic reaction in your baby, you won't know exactly which ingredient caused it.

Food Intolerance and Allergic Reactions

If your baby begins wheezing or develops rashes (including hives), a sore bottom, vomiting, or diarrhea after you've introduced a new food to her, she may have a food intolerance or be experiencing an allergic reaction. Allergic reactions are less common than food sensitivities or intolerances. Most food-allergy reactions are mild, but if your baby's reaction is severe or if you're unsure whether it's mild or severe, contact your baby's care provider or a health care professional immediately. If your baby has a mild reaction after eating a food, make sure you don't give her that food for several months. Then reintroduce it at first in very small amounts. (See Chapter 6 for more on food allergies.)

Common Sources of Food Allergies

Here's a list of the most common sources of food allergies in babies:

- Cow's milk
- Soy
- Egg whites
- Wheat
- Fish (such as tuna, salmon, and cod)
- Shellfish (such as shrimp, crab, and lobster)
- Nuts, especially tree nuts and peanuts (including peanut butter)

If you have a family history of allergies to any of these foods or your baby has severe eczema, talk with your baby's care provider before introducing them to your baby. Being at "high risk" for allergies is defined as having a parent or sibling with a documented allergic condition such as asthma, food allergy, allergic rhinitis, or eczema. Guidelines about the introduction of these foods to high-risk infants have changed. There is now some evidence to suggest that early introduction of these foods may indeed decrease the risk of allergy. It is currently recommended, if the introduction of other solid foods has gone well, to introduce a small taste of one of these foods at home (*not* at day care). If there is no obvious reaction, the food can be introduced in gradually increasing amounts.

Other Foods to Avoid

Avoid introducing the following foods to your baby for at least the first year of her life:

- Honey—this food is associated with infant botulism poisoning, a potentially deadly disease.
- Popcorn, whole nuts, seeds, hot dogs, raw carrots, whole grapes, chunks of apples, chunks of meats or cheese, hard candy, or any other food that she could choke on. These foods are best delayed until age three or four, as they are likely to cause choking.
- Heavily sweetened foods, like soda, lemonade, or baby-food desserts.
- Juices—giving babies plain water is a much healthier option than fruit juice, which offers no nutritional benefits over whole fruit and can contain added sugars.
- Cow's milk—it does not contain adequate iron. Yogurt and shredded cheese can be given.

Feeding Schedules

- At first, offer your baby a solid food once a day. Some parents find midmorning or midafternoon a better time than family mealtimes, because there's less distraction. *Note:* If your baby nurses but also eats lots of solids, she might not nurse as often or as long, which could consequently decrease your milk supply.
- After a couple of weeks, offer her solids twice a day.

- After about a month, start regularly offering her solids between nursing sessions or bottle feedings. At those times, your baby will have an appetite for solids but not be ravenous. Observe her appetite and satisfaction with what you're offering.
- Let your baby set the pace. She'll know when she's had enough food, just as she knows when she's had enough breast milk or formula. If you patiently let her set the pace, she'll gradually wean herself from the bottle or breast to solids. Also, try not to make your baby finish a portion. If you praise her for "cleaning her plate," she may polish off her food because she wants your approval, not because she's hungry.
- It's never too early to introduce the concept of family mealtime as a pleasant, social time of day to get together.

Age	Amounts of Food per Day
6–7 mos.	Breast milk or iron-fortified formula
	Pureed meats, fruits, and cooked vegetables (up to 8 tbs.)
	Iron-fortified single-grain cereal mixed with breast milk or formula (up to 8 tbs.)
8–9 mos.	Breast milk or iron-fortified formula
	Ground meat (and eggs if okayed by your care provider) (4 tbs.)
	Strained or finely chopped fruits and cooked vegetables (6–8 tbs.)
	Iron-fortified single-grain cereal mixed with breast milk or formula (8 tbs.)
10 mos. to 1 yr.	Breast milk or iron-fortified formula
	Chopped meat and other protein foods, like eggs (1–2 oz.)
	Mashed or bite-size fruits and cooked vegetables (6–8 tbs.)
	Iron-fortified cereal mixed with breast milk or formula (6–8 tbs.)
	Potato and whole-grain or enriched-grain products

This is just one example of a food plan. Many parents start with other foods or introduce foods in a different order.

How Much Food?

- At first, give your baby one to two teaspoons (5 to 10 milliliters) of food. Dilute the food with breast milk or formula.
- As her appetite grows and she becomes a more accomplished eater, gradually increase the amount to four to six tablespoons (59 to 89 milliliters). (A small jar of commercial baby food typically contains eight tablespoons—118 milliliters—of food.) Use the chart above as a guideline for your baby's first year.
- Again, never force your baby to eat, and don't make her eat "one last bite" when it's clear she's full.
- Your baby's behavior will tell you when she's full. She'll turn her head away from the spoon or close her lips tightly and refuse to take anything more into her mouth. Crying, gagging, or spitting out food may suggest your baby doesn't want more food, but these signs may also suggest that she hasn't learned how to eat solids.

How to Spoon Feed

From the time she was born, your baby knew how to eat only by sucking, so she may need time to learn how to eat from a spoon. To introduce spoon feeding, make sure your baby is sitting up, then place a small dab of food on the tip of a baby spoon. Place the spoon just between your baby's lips, and let her suck the food off it. Eventually, she'll take food from the spoon directly into her mouth.

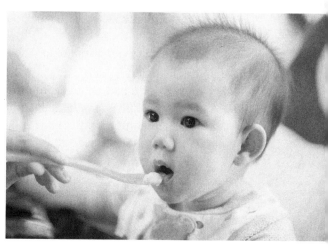

Messes

Babies learn about food by touching it, tasting it, and smelling it. This means, of course, that babies are messy eaters. The more you try to fight this fact, the more stressful mealtimes will be for you and your baby. Instead, relax and try to make mealtimes enjoyable, whatever the mess. If you want to make clean-up easier, place newspapers on the floor around where your baby eats. Wear an apron or clothes you don't mind getting stained, and put a bib on your baby.

What Kinds of Foods?

Your baby's first solid food could consist of a variety of options. Traditionally, a little iron-fortified single-grain cereal mixed with breast milk or formula has been the first solid food offered to American babies. Rice and oats are the most common grains—wheat should be introduced after six months of age. But recent studies suggest, especially for breastfed babies, that pureed meats (such as turkey, chicken, or beef) have the advantage of being rich in protein, iron, and zinc and thus have a higher nutrient value. Other cultures have traditionally offered foods such as avocado for the first solid. As your baby grows, her menu will expand but, as a general rule, meats and vegetables should be given some preference over fruits and cereals.

A Few Words about Juices

Contrary to popular belief, juice is *not* necessary to a baby's diet. In fact, drinking too much juice can lead to tooth decay, diarrhea, and diaper rash and can make your baby gain excess weight. If you do give your baby juice, make sure she's old enough to drink it from a cup and offer no more than four ounces a day. Make sure the juice is 100 percent juice, pasteurized and fortified with vitamin C, and not a "fruit drink." (You can water down the juices, but still don't offer your baby more than four ounces of diluted juice.) Make juice part of a snack, not part of a meal.

Vitamin Supplements

A balanced diet best ensures that your baby's getting the necessary vitamins. Once she starts eating a variety of solid foods, you might not need to give her any vitamin supplements, unless her care provider instructs otherwise. Check, in particular, about iron and vitamin D.

Stool Changes

You will surely notice a significant change in your baby's stools with the introduction of solids. They will have an odor, have a different color depending on which foods she consumes (they may be green after peas or red after beets, for example), and may contain undigested bits of food such as hulls of peas and corn, black strings from banana, and skins from tomatoes and other fruits and vegetables. Don't worry; this is normal.

Commercially Prepared Baby Foods

Commercially prepared baby foods are convenient and have been sterilized, and many contain vitamin and mineral supplements. Some manufacturers use organic foods. Most manufacturers have removed unnecessary additives, but still check the labels to make sure there's no added salt, sugar, or other preservatives or fillers (like flour or modified starch).

Here's a summary of the different commercially prepared baby foods:

- First Foods—six to seven months: Pureed, strained single-ingredient foods available in two-and-a-half-ounce portions. Use a spoon to introduce these foods (do not let your baby suck it out of a pouch).
- Second Foods—seven to eight months: Pureed combination food available in four-ounce jars.
- Third Foods—eight to ten months: Combination foods that often include milk and wheat and may contain spices; available in six-ounce jars.

Safe Feeding

Take all the precautions possible to keep your baby's food safe. Her immune system will need a couple of years to fully develop, so she'll be susceptible to bacterial growth. Here are a few things to remember when feeding your baby:

- Make sure your hands and all utensils used to prepare and serve your baby's food are clean.
- Don't feed your baby straight from a baby-food jar. Instead, spoon what you think she'll eat into a separate bowl and feed her from it. This will keep the bacteria in her mouth from being transferred to the jar and multiplying in the remaining food.
- Keep warm foods warm and cold foods cold. You should take the same precautions with your baby's food as you do with your own. Don't leave food out for more than one hour at room temperature. Refrigerate opened jars of food (as well as formula and breast milk) promptly.
- When your baby starts eating regular food or homemade baby food, make sure you cook it—especially meats—thoroughly.

Warming Baby Food

You don't need to warm your baby's food. In fact, she may prefer it at room temperature. If you warm the food, heat a jar of it in a pan of water on the stove or heat the food in a microwave set on low (stir well). Be very careful not to overheat it, and test the temperature of the food yourself before feeding it to your baby. Commercial baby-food warmers are also available.

Finger Food

When your baby is between eight and twelve months old, she'll probably want to start feeding herself. At this age, she's grown a few teeth and developed better hand coordination. Before you give her finger foods, she should be able to sit independently, grasp and release food, and chew and swallow food (even without teeth). Make sure that any finger foods you give her are soft, easy to swallow (or dissolve quickly in the mouth), and cut into bite-size pieces. Here's a list of nutritious finger foods that can be cut into small pieces and are appropriate for stomachs just getting used to solid foods:

- Shredded chicken and turkey
- Cooked egg yolks (whole eggs with whites may also be okay—check with your care provider)
- Hamburger pieces
- Finely diced beef, veal, and lamb
- Bits of low-mercury fish
- Tofu (soybean curd)
- Cooked beans
- Cooked pieces of apples, pears, and peaches
- Ripe bananas, avocado, mango, and melon
- Mashed potatoes and sweet potatoes
- Cooked peas, carrots, squash, cauliflower, and broccoli
- Cooked rice or lentils
- Macaroni, cooked very soft
- Sugarless dry cereal

Preparing Homemade Baby Foods

Many parents agree that homemade baby foods are often better than commercially prepared foods. For example, if you make your baby's food, you can do the following:

- Control more of what's in your baby's food
- Save money
- Protect the environment—no packaging to throw away
- Use organic produce and natural meats and poultry
- Provide more variety than what's available in commercially prepared baby foods
- Make foods that fit with your family's diet

You can quickly turn almost any of the foods you eat into something your baby will enjoy. All you need is something to grind the food. For example:

- Manual grinder: baby, small, or large food mill; fork; potato ricer; puree sieve; food chopper
- Electric grinder: blender; electric food mill; electric food chopper; electric mixer with attachments

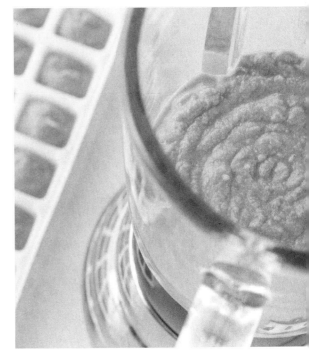

You also need something to store the baby food. Here are some inexpensive options:

- Ice cube trays: perfect for freezing baby food in small, individual portions
- Baking sheet: drop one- to two-tablespoon portions on a baking sheet and freeze.
- Small resealable plastic freezer bags: great for storing the frozen ice cubes, or "drops" of baby food and finger foods
- Small food-storage containers (less than three inches deep): can store baby food from the freezer to microwave

Tips for Preserving the Vitamins and Preparing Baby Food Safely

- Buy fresh produce no earlier than the day before you plan to prepare it.
- Keep produce at room temperature until peak ripeness.
- Wash your hands in hot soapy water before preparing food.
- Don't wash the food until you're ready to prepare it.

- Wash produce well, preferably with a produce rinse product, or a water and vinegar solution, to help remove pesticides.
- Use plastic or nonporous cutting boards. Wash them in hot soapy water after preparing each food item.
- Keep utensils and cutting boards used for raw meats, poultry, and fish separate from those used for raw fruit or vegetables.
- Chop food before cooking it to speed up cooking time.
- Steam or cook food either in the microwave with just a tablespoon of water or in a saucepan steamer rack.
- Don't add sugar, salt, or other seasonings while making baby food.
- Cook foods in small portions to prevent overcooking. Once cooked, refrigerate or freeze the portions after letting them cool briefly.
- Test the temperature of cooking meats with a food thermometer to make sure they're cooked properly.
- Wash knives, utensils, and countertops in hot soapy water after preparing each food item.
- Never place cooked food on a plate that held raw meat, poultry, or seafood. Avoid leaving any of these foods at room temperature.
- Make sure storage containers for baby food are clean.
- Use paper towels to clean up kitchen surfaces. If you must use cloth towels, wash them often in the hot cycle. If using sponges, wash them in the dishwasher and replace them often.

Homemade Baby Food Storage Guide		
Food	Refrigerator (40°F or 4°C)	Freezer (0°F or -18°C)
Cooked fruits and vegetables	2 days	1 mo.
Cooked meat, poultry, fish	24 hrs.	1 mo.
Frozen fruits and vegetables that have been thawed	2 days	Do not refreeze.
Cooked meat, poultry, or fish that has been thawed	24 hrs.	Do not refreeze.

Mercury in Fish

Fish is a high-quality protein that includes omega-3 fatty acids; it should be part of your baby's diet. Make sure to serve your baby fish that does not contain large amounts of mercury. Fish that are typically considered safe are shrimp, canned light tuna (vs. canned white or albacore), crab, salmon, tilapia, pollack, catfish, and freshwater trout. Fish that should be avoided are grouper, orange roughy, shark, swordfish, king mackerel, or tilefish. If the fish is caught fresh in a local lake or river, please check the mercury levels in that specific body of water; if you cannot, then limit that fish to one meal a week.

Preparing Baby Foods Step-by-Step

Step 1: Cook or steam the meats, fruits, or vegetables you plan to offer your baby. You can use canned fruits and vegetables, but they're not as nutritious as fresh or frozen foods.

Step 2: Puree, grind, mash, or finely chop the cooked foods. At first, make sure the food's texture is quite smooth. (Beginning eaters can choke on lumpy or coarse food.) The more experienced your baby becomes at eating, the less smooth her food's texture will need to be.

Step 3: Spoon the prepared food into an ice cube tray or onto a baking sheet, and freeze it. (Do not refreeze thawed foods.) When frozen, store the cubes or portions in resealable plastic freezer bags. Heat whatever amount you need in a pan on the stove or in the microwave.

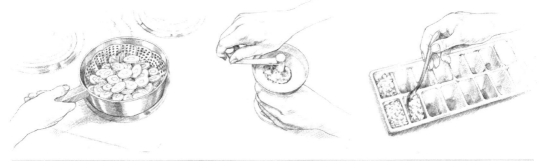

Pediatric Obesity

Almost one-third of children in the United States over two years of age are overweight. Issues such as genetic susceptibility, socioeconomic class, and geographic location have an impact on one's chances of being overweight, and researchers are still studying the specifics of what parents can do in the first year to prevent obesity, but here are a few logical steps you can take to start your child on a healthy path:

- Don't smoke during pregnancy. A recent study suggests that intrauterine exposure to smoke can be a risk for childhood obesity.
- Gain a healthy amount of weight during pregnancy. Women who gain too much may deliver babies with high birth weights, which could increase the risk for later obesity.
- Breastfeed, if possible. A breastfed baby is likely to be less obese through at least early adolescence.
- Wait to introduce solid foods until your baby is at least six months old.
- Allow your infant to stop eating at the earliest signs of being satisfied. Your role is to provide healthy, safe, and nutritious foods; your infant's role is to choose when and how much to eat.
- As your baby gets older, set a pattern of regular family mealtimes and snacks in a happy setting (with the TV, computer, and cell phones off).
- In your baby's first year (preferably two years) she should not have any foods or drinks that are high in sugar, sodium, and calories and low in nutrients, such as chips, cookies, carbonated soda, and fruit drinks.
- Don't put infant on a diet. Fat, particularly, should not be restricted in the first two years, since the brain is still growing.
- Bring your baby to her care provider for regular checkups. She or he will monitor growth rates (including length, weight, and head size) while factoring in familial patterns. You can help avoid overfeeding your baby by following the standardized growth charts from the World Health Organization (WHO). You and your care provider can work together to set the stage for good nutrition as well as physical activity that will bode well for the following years.

Chapter Four

Your Baby's Safety

Today's better health care has largely eliminated or controlled many diseases that once killed babies. In fact, vehicle accidents kill or injure more children under age four than any disease. As a parent, your job is to provide a safe environment that your baby can explore. Anticipate his development so you can childproof your home before he enters a new stage. And, of course, make sure he's properly secured in an approved car seat that is correctly installed in your car, when you travel.

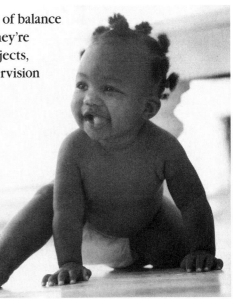

Babies are naturally curious and active, but their sense of balance and wariness of dangerous situations don't develop until they're older. Once your baby begins to wiggle, roll over, grasp objects, creep, and eventually crawl and walk, he'll need your supervision to explore his environment safely.

The following pages offer a guide to childproofing your home, plus information on buying safe baby equipment. At least every six months, childproof your home again. Focus on eliminating dangerous situations that your baby's drawn to. Also, consider the season—winter is an especially dangerous time for fires, and spring and summer often require water and bicycle safety precautions.

Here's a general outline of a baby's typical development during the first year (see Chapter 5 for details):

Age	Baby's Abilities
Birth–2 mos.	Your baby will wiggle and may start to roll over (though this is uncommon).
3–5 mos.	Your baby may begin to rock and roll over, grasp things, sit up, and put things into his mouth.
6–9 mos.	Your baby may begin to creep, crawl, pull himself up, and pull everything else down.
10–12 mos.	Your baby may begin to stand, climb, and even walk.

Childproofing Your Home

General Safety Guidelines

Here's a list of general home childproofing tips. Following them are tips for childproofing specific rooms and areas in your home.

- Cover unused outlets with safety caps. Use safety covers over outlets with electric plugs in them. Don't overload outlets. Make sure no electrical cords are frayed or damaged.

- Put bulbs in all empty light sockets.

- Don't let your baby near electrical appliances when they're in use, and always turn them off when you're done.

- Appliance cords, telephone cords, cords from blinds, and other cords or straps can strangle babies. Keep them out of your baby's reach. Any cords on toys should be shorter than seven inches, but watch your baby carefully when he's playing with any toy that has a cord.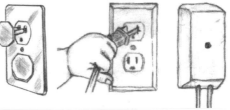

- Keep any objects that can fit inside a cardboard toilet paper tube out of your baby's reach (pins, buttons, screws, beads, coins, marbles, refrigerator magnets, small toys, and other small or sharp objects). It takes only a minute for a baby to put a small object in his mouth and choke. This warning also applies to any small, hard foods, like nuts or popcorn.

- Check your floors often for small objects, especially if you have older children who play with small toys or if you have a hobby that uses tiny materials.

- Keep scissors, knives, razor blades, tools, and all breakable or broken objects out of your baby's reach.

- Small button-cell batteries can cause severe injury and even death if ingested. Make sure batteries in remote controls, key fobs, greeting cards, and musical books are not accessible to your infant.

- Be aware and careful of what you put in your trash and where you keep your trash.

- Keep purses, briefcases, and bags out of your baby's reach. They often contain coins, sharp objects, medications, and other hazards.

- Keep all plastic bags and sheets of thin plastic out of your baby's reach. Dry cleaning bags are especially dangerous—tie them in a knot before throwing them away. Never cover a crib mattress with thin plastic.

- Never leave a baby alone with a balloon. Remove all popped-balloon pieces immediately so your baby doesn't choke on them.

- Never put necklaces, cords attached to pacifiers, or cords of any kind around your baby's neck.

- Keep your baby away from used ashtrays, glasses containing alcohol or hot liquids, lit candles, matches, or cigarette lighters—these last two items are the most common cause of fatal fires.

- Don't smoke while caring for your baby. Cigarettes can burn him, and the smoke can irritate his lungs and make him more susceptible to diseases. *Never* smoke in bed.

- Install smoke and carbon monoxide detectors in your basement and in the hallways near bedrooms. Make sure you have at least one smoke detector on each floor of your home or on both ends of a mobile home. Never apply paint over a smoke or carbon monoxide detector. Test all smoke detectors monthly, replace batteries yearly, replace all smoke detectors every ten years, and all carbon monoxide detectors every five to seven years. Vacuum or dust them regularly. If there are members of a household that are hard of hearing, make sure the detectors have a flashing-light mechanism to provide a visual alert.

- Your children should wear clothing made with naturally flame-retardant cloth (like polyester or fleece) to bed; if you must use clothing that isn't flame retardant, make sure it fits snugly so there's little air between the fabric and your baby's skin. (Air feeds a flame if the fabric is on fire.)

- Have a fire escape plan and practice it monthly. Make sure windows and doors can open easily. Plan for two ways to be able to exit each room.

- In the event of a fire, test any closed doors for heat before deciding whether to open them. Crawl low under the smoke to get away from the fire and do not go back under any circumstances. Remember the "Stop, Drop, and Roll" rule for anyone who catches fire and to apply anything cool to the skin immediately after this.

- Be up to date on the weather-related risk factors where you live, including hurricanes, tornadoes, flash floods, and earthquakes. Learn how best to protect yourself and your child in the event of such a disaster.

- Place guards in front of open fireplaces, heaters, steam radiators, hot-air registers, floor furnaces, and riser pumps. Have your furnace, fireplaces, and chimney cleaned and inspected yearly. Avoid using electric space heaters or kerosene heaters. If you must use them, keep them away from bedding, clothing, and curtains. Unplug them at night.

- Firearms should not be kept in homes with infants and children. If, despite this warning, they are, always store guns unloaded and firearms and ammunition locked up separately.

- Remove furniture with sharp edges from rooms where your baby crawls around. Soft plastic safety edges are great for covering sharp corners on coffee tables and other low furniture. You can also use foam tape to cover the edges of glass tables.

- Be aware of dangers associated with doors, especially transparent glass doors that can be run into, swinging doors that can knock one down, and folding doors that can pinch fingers. Removal of these doors may be the safest option. Try to open windows from the top, if possible. Regardless, make sure a lock prevents falling out of windows.

- If you have hardwood floors, don't allow your child to walk or run on them in socks or booties without slip-resistant soles.

- Some large-screen TVs, bookcases, and computer monitors can fall over, seriously harming or even killing those crushed. Consider installing wall tethers to heavy pieces of furniture.

- If your home's walls, windows, or doors were last painted before 1977, consider repainting. Old paint contains lead that can harm your baby, especially if he eats any paint chips. You can find devices to check for lead at some paint stores or home improvement centers. If repainting, follow the Environmental Protection Agency's guidelines for safely removing lead-based paint (see http://www.epa.gov/lead/pubs/renovaterightbrochure.pdf).

Kitchen or Dining Room

- Keep toxic materials (see page 115) locked up or out of your baby's reach. Use drawer and cupboard safety latches to prevent him from getting into potentially dangerous items. Dishwasher detergent pods contain very concentrated chemicals that can be poisonous and must be kept locked in a secure location.

- Make sure your baby can't get into any garbage pails or wastebaskets.

- If possible, have someone else care for your baby in another room while you're cooking and serving meals, or use a high chair or play yard to keep your child away from danger. Hot grease and food can splatter a baby sitting nearby in a baby carrier, and a mobile baby can get into lots of danger.

- Turn all pot handles inward so your baby can't pull them off the stove. Simmer foods on the front burners and boil foods on the back burners. Keep anything that could catch fire away from the stove and oven.

- Never leave the oven door open, and keep your baby away from oven doors that are hot to the touch. If possible, keep your infant out of the kitchen entirely when the oven is on.

- Don't let your baby play with knobs on a gas stove. If necessary, remove the knobs when you're not using them.

- Don't drink hot liquids while your baby's in your lap. When carrying hot liquids, make sure you don't trip over your baby or anything that could cause a spill onto your child.

- Keep all objects away from the edges of counters and tables, out of your baby's reach.

- Unplug appliances when not in use.

- Sharp knives and appliances such as food processors should be kept in latched drawers or cupboards.

- Avoid putting small magnets on the outside of your refrigerator. They're a choking hazard.

- Keep matches out of sight and reach.

- Avoid using tablecloths. Babies love to pull on the edges and can pull objects onto themselves.
- Install a multipurpose, dry-chemical, portable fire extinguisher in the kitchen. Know when and how you should use it.

Bathroom

- Never leave your baby alone in the bathtub—not even for a second.
- Before bathing your baby, always make sure the bathwater isn't too hot. Turn off the faucets tightly so your baby can't turn them on. Set your hot water heater to 120°F (48.9°C) so your baby won't be unintentionally scalded.
- Always keep the bathroom door closed, and don't let your baby play in the bathroom. A bathroom contains too many hard objects and slippery surfaces, and a curious child could drown in a toilet bowl. Consider installing a lock on the toilet seat cover.
- Keep hot curling irons and electric razors well away from your baby. Unplug and put away hairdryers when they're not in use, especially if they're near any source of water.
- Put away medicines and other potentially hazardous materials—cleansers, cosmetics, and soaps (see page 115)—immediately after use. Store them in a locked, high cabinet out of reach.
- Buy medicine in childproof containers and store them in locked cabinets.
- Always check medicine labels in a well-lit room for proper dosages before administering medications to your baby. Don't give medications prescribed for one baby to another.
- Don't save leftover medications; safely discard them.
- Don't call medicine and supplements "candy." Many poisonings are overdoses of good-tasting medicine and supplements, like candy-flavored vitamins.

Nursery

- Never leave your baby alone on a changing table, bed, couch, or other elevated surface. While changing your baby, use a safety strap or keep one hand on him at all times. If you must leave the room in the middle of a diaper change, take him with you or lay him in a crib or other safe place.
- Buy only clothing made from naturally flame-retardant cloth (like polyester or fleece) for your baby. If you must use clothing that isn't flame retardant, make sure it fits snugly so there's little air between the fabric and your baby's skin. (Air feeds a flame if the fabric is on fire.)
- When your baby can sit up by himself, lower the crib mattress. Set it at its lowest point before he can stand.
- Don't have bumper pads, blankets, or stuffed toys in your baby's crib.
- Place humidifiers, vaporizers, and portable heaters out of your child's reach, and keep them away from his bedding and anything else flammable.

- Contact your local fire department to learn what fire safety measures it recommends. If the nursery isn't on the ground floor, make sure you've got a fire escape plan that provides a safe way to reach the ground. Buy a noncombustible escape ladder, if necessary.
- Install window guards to prevent falls.

Stairs

- To prevent falls while carrying your baby as you walk up and down a staircase, keep all objects off the stairs. Remove extension cords and throw rugs near or on the staircase. Hold the handrail while climbing up or down. Carpet your stairs if possible. Don't wax uncarpeted stairs.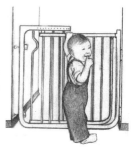
- When your baby is mobile, barricade the tops and bottoms of staircases with safety gates that are mounted to the wall (pressure gates aren't as sturdy). Babies learn to climb up before they learn to climb down. Any gaps should be less than one and a half inches (3.8 centimeters) wide.
- If you have a basement door, install a self-latching lock to prevent falls down the stairs.

Laundry

- Store all laundry detergents and cleaning products out of your child's reach. Laundry detergent pods are particularly dangerous because of the concentration of the chemicals and must be locked in a secure place.
- Clean your dryer lint trap after every use and the vent every year to avoid lint buildup that can catch fire.
- Don't let your baby near your iron or ironing board; an ironing board is easily tipped over, and an iron is hot, heavy, and easily pulled down by tugging on the cord. Always turn the iron off when you're done.
- Tie dry cleaning bags in a knot before throwing them away.

Outdoors

- Don't bring your baby—or any child—in the yard when you're using lawnmowers, snowblowers, or any power equipment. Never ride with or carry your baby when you're operating this equipment.
- Never leave your baby alone outside.
- Make sure your baby doesn't pick up dangerous objects or put them in his mouth.
- Your baby needs some sun exposure to stimulate the production of vitamin D, which is necessary for building strong bones. Two to three times a week during the warmer months, expose some of your baby's skin (hands, arms, and face) to sunlight for five to fifteen minutes. If your baby has darker skin, have him sunbathe slightly longer. To prevent burning at other times, place a wide-brimmed hat on your baby's head and, until he's six months old, dress him in as much clothing as is comfortable and lightly apply a PABA-free sunblock (at least SPF 15) on his hands and face. Once he's six months old,

slather sunblock on any exposed skin. Midday sunlight is the strongest, so expose your baby to the sun before 10 a.m. and after 4 p.m.

- Use and store barbecue grills away from anything flammable. Use grills outside only, and don't place them against the wall of your home. Make sure your child can't touch the grill. Charcoal should be cold before it is dumped.

- Always place barriers around fire pits or campfires. Constantly supervise your child around an outdoor fire. Make sure the fire is completely out before leaving it.

- Store gasoline, kerosene, and propane away from your home and only in approved safety containers.

- If pesticides or herbicides are applied to your yard, keep your child away from the yard for at least forty-eight hours.

Toxic Substances

- Post the phone number of the national poison control center (800-222-1222) near every telephone and program it into your cell phone(s). Consider also posting and programming the phone number of your local poison control center.

- If your baby has swallowed a substance, call the poison control center. Get to a medical facility as soon as possible, if recommended. (See pages 200–201.) Do *not* give your baby syrup of Ipecac.

- If your baby has a substance in his eye, hold his eyelid open and pour a steady stream of lukewarm water into the inner corner of the eye. If a substance is on his skin, remove clothing and rinse the skin with lukewarm water.

- If your baby may have been exposed to toxic fumes, get him to a safe location away from the fumes immediately, and contact the local poison center for further guidance.

- Keep all toxic substances in a locked container and stored in a drawer or cupboard, out of your baby's reach. Keep the drawer or cupboard closed and use safety latches to prevent your baby from opening it.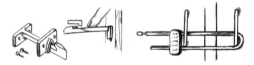

- Keep all toxic substances in their original containers with their original labels.

- Discard containers that have held hazardous substances into a garbage pail with a locked lid, or remove them from your home.

- Don't let your baby chew on newspaper, magazine, or book pages. Some inks may be toxic.

- Don't let your baby chew on gift-wrap ribbons. The dye in some ribbons may be toxic.

- Don't let your child chew on windowsills, porch steps, bars on iron gates, or any other surfaces. They may have been painted with lead-based paint.

- Don't take medication or supplements in front of your baby. If he wants to put everything into his mouth that you put into yours, he may find your medications and supplements attractive.

Environmental Concerns

The list of potentially toxic materials in the environment is growing. These include substances like radon, asbestos, formaldehyde, mercury, molds, lead, water contaminants, and many more chemicals. Keep a diligent watch for updated information on these types of substances. (The Environmental Protection Agency's website is a helpful resource: http://www.epa.gov/. You can also find specialized pediatric environmental health information at http://www.pehsu.net.)

Following is a general list of household products and other potentially poisonous substances. Many others may be poisonous as well. If you question whether a substance is poisonous, ask your baby's care provider or call the poison control center.

• Alcoholic beverages • Ammonia • Antifreeze • Aspirin, vitamins containing iron, and other drugs and medicines • Bleach • Borax • Car cleaner • Cleaning products (fluids and powders) • Cosmetics	• Detergents, including detergent pods • Drain cleaners • E-cigarette liquid nicotine • Furniture polish • Hair relaxer • Insect and rat poisons • Kerosene, gasoline, and benzene • Lamp oil • Lead-based paint	• Liquid furniture and car polish • Lighter fluid • Lye and alkalies for cleaning drains, toilet bowls, and ovens • Metal polish • Mothballs • Mouthwash • Nail products • Oil of wintergreen • Paint thinner	• Perfumes • Perm solutions • Pesticides • Plant sprays and weed killers • Rust remover • Shoe polish • Toilet bowl cleaners • Turpentine • Washing soda • Wax remover • Windshield washer fluid

Poisonous Plants

Many household and garden plants are poisonous—you might not want to keep plants in your home. Otherwise, know the names of all your plants, and keep them out of your baby's reach. Never let him eat or suck on any part of a plant. Nibbling on leaves, sucking on plant stalks, or drinking and eating from a surface where plants have been may poison him.

Following is a partial list of poisonous plants; there are many more. There are also many plants that are mildly toxic. Contact the national poison control center (800-222-1222) or your local poison control center for a more complete list of toxic plants.

• Azalea • Crocus (autumn) • Delphinium • Elderberry • Holly	• Hydrangea • Japanese yew • Larkspur • Lily of the valley • Marijuana	• Mistletoe • Morning glory • Nightshade • Oleander • Poison ivy	• Poison oak • Poison sumac • Rhododendron • Toadstools • Wisteria

Baby Gear

This section outlines the most common, helpful baby gear. Here are a few general safety tips to remember about baby gear:

- Mail all completed product registration and warranty cards so you're notified of manufacturer recalls.
- If you buy or receive used baby gear, always check online for recalls, and look over the gear for cracks, overuse, or missing pieces. When in doubt, do not use it.
- Check the Consumer Product Safety Commission website for recalls and up-to-date product information at http://www.cpsc.gov.

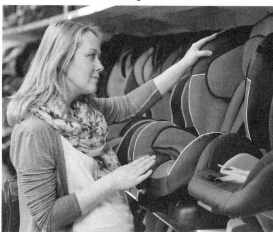

- For more information on product safety and quality, read a current product ratings guide, like *Consumer Reports* (http://www.consumer reports.org).
- Check that all new baby gear has a certification safety seal from the Juvenile Products Manufacturers Association (JPMA).
- Don't place any gear directly under ceiling fans, by heating elements, windows, or electrical cords.

Car Seat

As mentioned previously, vehicle accidents injure or kill more children younger than age four than any other kind of accident or disease. For this reason, it's illegal for children to ride in vehicles without being strapped into car seats. Most crashes occur within five miles (8 kilometers) of home at speeds of less than twenty-five miles (40 kilometers) per hour, so always use the car seat no matter how short your ride. State laws vary on what age children must be before they can travel without them, and car seat weight and height limits differ by model.

Car seats reduce the chance (by well over 95 percent) that your baby will be harmed or killed in a vehicle accident. When a vehicle hits an object or stops suddenly, everyone inside continues to move forward at the same speed at which the vehicle was traveling—and restraints prevent them from becoming flying projectiles. You can't protect your baby while traveling in a vehicle by holding him snugly in your arms. Even if you're wearing a seat belt, the force of a crash will tear your baby from your arms. And if you strap your baby in with you, a crash will slam your own weight into his body, causing serious or fatal injuries. Car seats are designed to spread the force of a crash evenly over a baby's body.

Most hospitals and birth centers won't let you drive your baby home if you don't have a federally approved car seat that's properly installed. For guidelines on buying a car seat, check the Consumer Reports website at http://www.consumerreports.org. To make sure the car seat is safely installed, have a certified child passenger safety (CPS) technician check it. These experts can be located by entering your state and zip code at http://www.seatcheck.org or by calling 1-866-seat-check. The National Highway Traffic Safety Administration is another resource and can be accessed by telephone at 888-DASH-2-DOT (888-327-4236) from 8 a.m. to 10 p.m. (eastern standard time) Monday through Friday or online at http://www.nhtsa.dot.gov; click on the car seat link.

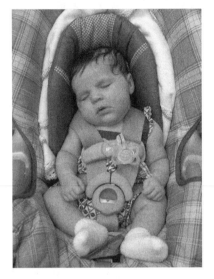

- Read your vehicle owner's manual for important information on how to install a car seat correctly in your vehicle. For individual help installing a specific car seat in a specific car, consult a certified child passenger safety (CPS) technician.
- All babies must be in a rear-facing car seat for the entire first year.
- Install the car seat in the back seat, preferably in the center.
- Never put a rear-facing car seat in the front seat of a car with an airbag.
- Use the correct harness slots for your baby's size.
- Place the plastic harness clip at or below your baby's shoulder level to hold shoulder straps in place.
- Make sure the straps lie flat and aren't twisted. Adjust the straps to accommodate the thickness of your baby's clothes, checking that the harness still holds him snugly.
- If your baby's head slumps forward, the seat might not be reclined enough. Tilt the car seat until it's reclined as close as possible to a forty-five-degree angle (according to manufacturer's instructions). You can place a rolled towel or other firm padding such as a pool noodle under the base of the seat near the point where the back and bottom of the vehicle seat meet.
- Dress your baby in clothes that allow the car seat straps between his legs.
- In cold weather, tuck blankets around your baby *after* securing and adjusting the harness straps.
- Pad the sides of the seat and between your baby's legs with rolled-up receiving blankets or a small diaper to keep your newborn from slouching.
- If your infant is premature or very small, he should be observed in the car seat while still in the hospital to make sure the semireclined position doesn't lower his heart rate or oxygen level or cause other breathing problems. If your child has special needs, he may need a car seat that's custom designed for his situation.
- Don't attach anything to a car seat, even educational baby toys. Attached items could pose a danger in an accident.

- All built-in child seats are for children at least a year old and who weigh at least twenty pounds.
- Don't use a car seat in a boat. They don't float.
- Don't transport unsecured heavy or loose objects while traveling with your baby in a vehicle.
- Never leave your baby alone in a vehicle—not even for a minute.

Crib

A crib can be your child's bed until age two or older.

- The safest place for an infant to sleep is in a crib with a firm mattress with a well-fitted sheet.
- Make sure to lower the mattress when your baby can sit up, and put the mattress in the lowest position before he can stand.
- Purchase a new crib, if possible. Older cribs might not meet current safety standards. If you must use an older or secondhand crib, check it carefully for potential hazards, replace the mattress, and check the Consumer Product Safety Commission website (http://www.cpsc.gov) for any recalls on the crib. Also, never pass a used crib to a new family without checking for recalls.
- Cribs with detachable drop-side rails, corner posts (finials), and large cutouts on the headboard and footboard have all been recalled for strangulation hazards. Do not use any crib that has these.
- Make sure there are no missing, loose, cracked, or splintered slats, no sharp or jagged edges.
- Check that the space between slats is no more than two and three-quarters inches (6 centimeters) wide to prevent your baby's head from becoming trapped.
- Check that the mattress fits snugly in the crib. (No more than two fingers should fit between the edge of the mattress and the side of the crib.) Remove any plastic covering the mattress.
- Make sure the screws or bolts holding crib parts together are tight and none are missing to prevent the crib from coming apart. Recheck often that parts are tight fitting, and only replace parts with ones from the manufacturer.
- Don't place any bumper pads, pillows, comforters, blankets, stuffed animals, or other soft items in the crib because of the potential risk of suffocation, strangulation, or entrapment.
- Use sleep sacks or footed pajamas instead of a blanket to keep your baby warm.
- Make sure that mobiles are securely attached to the side rails and the hanging items on mobiles aren't long enough to strangle your baby. Once your baby is five months old (or mobile), remove crib gyms and hanging mobiles from the crib.
- Don't hang things with strings or ribbons in the crib.

- Don't place the crib near blinds, draperies, or electrical cords to prevent strangulation.
- Don't place the crib near a window.
- When the height of the side rail is less than three-quarters of your baby's height, his height reaches thirty-five inches (89 centimeters), or he is trying to climb out of the crib, move him to a bed.

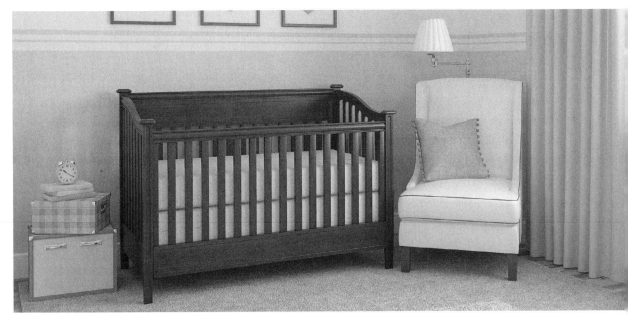

Bassinet or Cradle

Bassinets and cradles are small cribs that an infant can sleep in for their first month. Typically they are used in the parents' room to keep an infant close for bonding and feeding and are meant to meet the American Academy of Pediatrics (AAP) guidelines for sudden infant death (SIDS) prevention, which suggest it's best for an infant to sleep in the same room but not the same bed as his parents.

Stroller

Choosing the right stroller depends on your lifestyle. In general, look for a stroller with buckles and belts that are easy to fasten and adjust, an adjustable seat and canopy, washable fabric, an adjustable handle, an easy folding mechanism with a safety catch, brakes, wide wheel base, and swivel wheels.

Baby Carrier Packs (Backpacks and Front Packs)

A wearable carrier lets you transport your baby either in or outside the house and keeps your hands free to do other tasks. To be safe, pick a carrier that fits your baby's height, weight, and age. (Check the manufacturer's specifications.)

Bouncer Seat, Baby Swing, Play Center, Play Yard, and Jumper

A bouncer seat, baby swing, stationary play center, or a baby jumper can be helpful if you need time to do chores or other activities that require your baby to be away from you (like cooking dinner, taking a shower, scrubbing a toilet, or taking a moment for yourself). Don't rely on any of them too much (no more than fifteen to thirty minutes); nothing can replace your loving touch and lots of unrestricted playtime. Your baby needs to explore his environment to develop his motor and balance skills; don't substitute a play yard for a properly childproofed home.

High Chair

Once your baby starts to eat solid foods and can sit up on his own—usually between six and eight months—he'll need a place to sit so you can feed him easily. Make sure to use the safety straps properly, and never let your baby stand up in the high chair.

Changing Table

A changing table can be a convenient place to dress your baby and change his diaper in the first few months. Never leave your baby alone on a changing table or other elevated surface. While changing your baby, use a safety strap or keep one hand on him at all times. If you must leave the room in the middle of a diaper change, take him with you or lay him in a crib or other safe place. See pages 29–30 for more information on changing tables.

Baby Monitor

A baby monitor lets you listen to or see your baby from another room. It will help you know if your baby needs to be fed, changed, or comforted—all while giving you the freedom to do things outside the nursery. Place the baby monitor at least ten feet from your baby's crib (and turn it off when it's not needed) to help minimize any potential EMF radiation.

Other Safety Issues

General Car Safety

When your baby is old enough to be mobile, keep him away from driveways and streets where he may be hit by a vehicle. Drivers should always walk around and behind their vehicles before getting in to make sure no one is in the blind spot.

Bicycle Seats

Bicycle seats aren't recommended for babies during the first year. It's also not safe to ride a bicycle with your baby in a front pack or backpack. Even a ride in a bicycle-towed trailer before one year of age can jar your baby's body too much. Trailers can be dangerous to use on roadways as they are low and motorists might not see them. Once your baby is a year old and his neck can support a bicycle helmet, a bicycle trailer is still a safer way than a bicycle seat to take him for a ride.

Boating and Life Jackets

If you include your baby in your family's water activities, make sure he wears an appropriate personal floatation device (PFD) that's been approved by the United States Coast Guard. Follow the weight guidelines for the PFD, and make sure your baby will float in an upright position if he gets into the water. For a younger baby, it must have a floatation collar. The PFD must fit properly, and you should not be able to lift it over your baby's head. Never use inflatable toys and rings as life preservers. Make sure you and everyone else on a watercraft wear life jackets; in case of an accident, you'll need to be able to assist your baby. Never strap your baby into a car seat while in a boat; car seats do not float.

Shopping Carts

Every year, falls from shopping carts seriously injure children. To keep your baby safe, use all the safety straps for built-in seats.

If using your own seat, place it completely in the cart. Don't balance it on the edges. Never let your baby ride unrestrained, and constantly keep an eye on him while he's in the cart.

Before you place your baby into a cart, use a sanitizing wipe on the handles and seat to protect him from germs. Many stores now provide wipes, but consider keeping a small supply in your purse or diaper bag.

Pet Safety

- Before your new baby arrives, think about spaying or neutering your pets; this makes them calmer and less likely to bite. You should also address any behavior problems they may have, and clip their nails or claws.
- Once your baby is born, have your partner or a family member take something with your baby's scent (a blanket, for example) home, to familiarize your pet with it.
- Always supervise your baby when he's in a room with animals. Watch your pet for any aggressive or defensive behaviors.
- Once your baby is crawling, make sure to keep pet food and pet toys out of his reach.
- If you plan to get a new dog, do research beforehand. Certain breeds (Rottweilers, German shepherds, and pit bulls) are less family friendly.
- Reptiles can cause salmonella infections in children. Your child should not have contact with any lizards, turtles, or snakes until he is five years old.

Traveling

Traveling with your baby usually takes some planning (sometimes a *lot* of planning), but it can be done and often with minimal fuss. The key is to plan ahead while staying flexible. To keep your baby calm and content during any trip, dress him appropriately and bring along toys, snacks (if he's eating solid foods), and plenty of diapers. On a road trip, know that you'll need to stop more often than you otherwise would, for feedings and diaper changes.

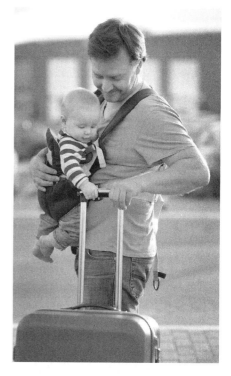

Before a trip, especially a lengthy one, talk with your baby's health care provider about where you'll be traveling and for how long. It's important that your baby keeps to his vaccination schedule, and you may need to work the trip around the schedule (or vice versa). Check what medical facilities are available at your destination in case your baby requires medical attention. Bring along a first-aid kit, any medications your baby may need to take, and your baby's care provider's contact information.

Air Travel

According to the Federal Aviation Administration (FAA), parents don't have to buy seats for children younger than age two. Instead, parents can carry their babies on their laps. This less expensive option may sound tempting, but it's much safer for your baby to travel in his own seat while sitting in his car seat.

Any currently manufactured car seat approved for use on an airplane must have an FAA approval label. If you plan to fly on a smaller commercial plane, check with the airline to make sure your baby's car seat will fit in the airplane seat. Typically, a seat whose base is less than sixteen inches (40.6 centimeters) wide will fit in most coach seats. Properly secure the car seat to the airline seat and strap your baby in correctly. Make sure his height and weight don't exceed the car seat's recommended limit.

If you use a car seat on an airplane, book adjacent seats ahead of time for you and your baby. A car seat must be placed in a window seat that's not in an emergency exit row—this is so it won't block your (or another passenger's) movement in an emergency.

If you want to save money but also want to try to have your baby ride in his car seat, take the seat with you to the gate. Your flight might not be full, and you can ask to be assigned next to one of the unassigned seats and use it to secure your baby's car seat (if, of course, either seat is next to a window and neither is in an emergency exit row). Try to book a flight at an off-peak time to increase your chances of getting an empty seat. If you learn at the gate that the flight is full, check the car seat. Make sure you and your baby aren't assigned to a row with another "lap baby"; in an emergency, there will be only one extra oxygen mask for each row. Don't strap your baby into the seat belt with you; instead, strap yourself in and hold on to him.

Here are some other tips for air travel with your baby:

- An umbrella stroller works well for air travel. You can use it in airports, and it can fold up and fit in an overhead compartment.
- Nurse your baby (or give him a bottle or pacifier) during takeoff and landing. Sucking and swallowing will equalize the air pressure in his ears.
- If you plan to travel with expressed breast milk, the TSA recommends you declare the breast milk before screening and carry a printout of this web page (http://www.tsa.gov /traveling-formula-breast-milk-and-juice) to help prevent problems at security checkpoints.
- Consider beforehand your baby's feeding schedule during the flight and pack any necessary equipment (for example, a blanket for privacy during breastfeeding or extra water-filled bottles and powdered formula). If your child is eating solid foods, choose foods that aren't messy or can be easily cleaned up. Keep in mind that flights are often delayed and you may need to prepare for extra feedings.
- Pack a change of clothes for your baby in your carry-on luggage. If he spits up or his diaper leaks, you'll be ready with a fresh outfit.
- Remember to bring small toys to entertain your baby. Make sure, however, that the toys won't annoy other passengers, especially if they're trying to sleep.
- In general, try to pack anything in your carry-on luggage that you wouldn't want to be left without during the flight: baby wipes, diapers, a favorite toy, and so on.
- Some airplane restrooms have changing tables, but many don't. If you need to change your baby's diaper at your seat, put the soiled diaper into an airsickness bag and toss it into the restroom trash.

Other Safety Tips

- If you're staying in a hotel, find out whether babyproofing equipment will be available. If not, bring your own (including electrical outlet covers, door latches for bathrooms and minibars, covers for sharp-edged furniture, and safety gates if you're staying in a room with a balcony). Check the hotel floor to be sure there are no small objects your baby could put into his mouth. Bring your own play yard for your baby to sleep in. If you need to rent a crib, make sure you reserve it beforehand, and look it over carefully before placing your baby in it.
- If you're traveling in a car, always use a car seat in the correct position. Place a wide-brimmed hat on your baby or use shade screens on the windows to keep him cool and safe from sun exposure. Never leave your baby alone in a car.
- If traveling by bus or train, bring along your baby's car seat. There might not be safety belts to secure the seat, but your baby will be more protected in his seat than in your lap.

Chapter Five

Your Baby's Development

A baby's first year is an exciting time for parents. During this period, your baby changes from a helpless newborn to an active toddler who explores, communicates, solves problems, and begins to assert her independence in many ways. This transformation brings new experiences to you and your baby and lets you both develop new skills.

Although children usually develop skills in the same sequence, each child learns them on her own schedule. For example, your baby may learn to crawl earlier than other babies, but she may learn to hold a spoon later. She should eventually learn all the skills she's supposed to, and she'll spend the first year practicing and perfecting the skills she's already learned.

Developmental screening is one part of your baby's routine well-child checkups. Your child's health care provider will let you know if your baby is meeting her milestones and may ask you to complete a questionnaire specific to your baby's age. Let the provider know if you have any questions about your baby's development.

All healthy children have an instinctual urge to learn, explore, and grow. Provide your baby a safe, interesting environment for her to discover, and limit her activity as little as possible (while still keeping her safe, of course). You probably won't need to formally teach her skills at this age,

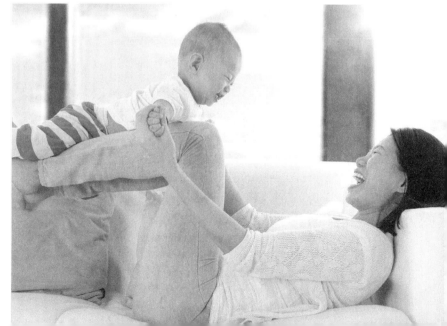

but interact with her as much as possible. She'll learn from the games she'll naturally play with you and from your actions that she'll eventually imitate. Observe her preferences and attempts to initiate interaction. Learn her cues and respond to them. As your baby grows, she'll try new ways to learn more complex skills.

This chapter presents a baby's typical milestones of development during the first year. Keep in mind that skills don't develop according to a strict timeline. In most cases, there's no reason to worry if your baby strays from the schedule during the first year.

Developmental milestones are often subdivided into categories such as physical, social/emotional, and sensory. Further subcategories includes gross motor, fine motor, self-help, cognitive, and receptive and expressive language skills.

Note: If you have a premature baby, she might need more time to reach certain milestones. Her health care provider will likely use her adjusted age (her age based on her due date, rather than her birth date) to assess her development. Don't worry; she'll probably catch up to other children by the time she's two or three.

Developmental Milestones Month-by-Month

	Gross Motor	Fine Motor	Cognitive	Language	Social	Warning Signs
First Month	Makes reflex movements (e.g., grasping or stepping) Turns chin up when on stomach Brings hands near face Can move head side to side when on back	Strong grip Hands fisted Sucks well	Sleeps a lot and will be alert for only brief times each day Stares at hands and fingers Prefers looking at faces and patterns with contrasting colors Comforts herself by mouthing and sucking her fist and fingers	Hears very well Recognizes some sounds, including parents' voices	Tracks movement with eyes Makes eye-to-eye contact at close range, usually eight to twelve inches away from you Shows enjoyment by quieting down and possibly smiling briefly Distinguishes one or two people by their voices	Sucks poorly and feeds slowly Doesn't react to bright lights or loud sounds Doesn't focus and follow a nearby object moving side to side Rarely moves arms and legs Seems especially stiff or floppy Lower jaw trembles constantly, even when not crying or excited

	Gross Motor	Fine Motor	Cognitive	Language	Social	Warning Signs
Second Month	Holds up head and neck briefly while on tummy Begins to push up when lying on tummy Makes smoother movements with arms and legs Rolls from side to side Lies with one arm straight out, her head turned to that side, and the other arm flexed up (the "fencing" position)	Opens and closes hands Begins to play with fingers Begins to control her grasp and holds an object for a few minutes	Pays attention to faces or moving objects but can only focus on close objects Begins to follow things with her eyes and recognizes people at a distance Begins to act bored (cries, fussy) if activity doesn't change Uses only one sense at a time (e.g., sucking in bursts, then looking around during pauses) Opens mouth at sight of breast or bottle	Coos and makes gurgling sounds Turns head toward sounds	Smiles responsively Can briefly calm herself Recognizes her primary caregiver's voice and touch Connects some positions and people with certain events—for instance, her mother with feeding Begins to seek and respond to attention by smiling, making sounds, and actively moving her arms and legs	Doesn't respond to loud sounds Doesn't watch things as they move Doesn't smile at people Doesn't bring hands to mouth Can't hold head up when pushing up while on tummy
Third Month	Reaches and grabs at objects Rests on her forearms when lying on her stomach and holding her head up Sits supported for a few minutes Stretches legs out and kicks when lying on stomach or back Pushes down on legs when feet are placed on a firm surface	Opens and shuts hands Grabs and shakes hand toys Brings hands to mouth Begins to reach for an object with both hands Bats at things and kicks with force	Explores a room for light, colors, shapes, and patterns, and searches for a sound source Looks and sucks at the same time Can be attentive for up to forty-five minutes at a time Begins to show memory of sequences, effects, and people Uses various movements and expressions to show her moods and needs Starts using hands and eyes in coordination	Makes sounds in response to talking and singing	Imitates you when you stick out your tongue Smiles spontaneously Recognizes familiar objects and people at a distance Watches faces closely, imitates some movements and facial expressions Enjoys playing with other people and may cry when playing stops	Cannot support her head well Has trouble moving one or both eyes in all directions Crosses her eyes most of the time (Occasional crossing of the eyes is normal in these first months.) Doesn't pay attention to new faces, or seems very frightened by new faces or surroundings Doesn't smile at people Doesn't follow moving objects with her eyes Doesn't grasp objects

	Gross Motor	Fine Motor	Cognitive	Language	Social	Warning Signs
Fourth Month	Splashes in the bath Rolls from back to side or from stomach to side or back Sits supported, with her head steady, for ten to fifteen minutes When lying on stomach, pushes up to elbows	Reaches for toy with one hand Grabs objects—gets them! Looks at and plays with her hands Puts everything in her mouth Can hold a toy and shake it Swings at dangling toys	Turns her head and eyes to look in all directions Watches moving people Can locate a sound source Becomes attached to an object or toy Is alert for at least one hour at a time and has sustained interest in details Increases her activity when she anticipates a feeding Enjoys eating as a social and play time May no longer need a night feeding	Laughs out loud Begins to babble with expression Copies sounds she hears Cries in different ways to show hunger, pain, or tiredness Copies some movements and facial expressions, like smiling or frowning	Discriminates among faces and knows her primary caregiver Smiles spontaneously, especially at people Responds to affection	Doesn't babble Doesn't bring objects to her mouth Can't hold head steady Doesn't push down with her legs when her feet are placed on a firm surface Doesn't watch things as they move
Fifth Month	Can be easily pulled to standing Moves by rocking, rolling (from stomach to back or back to side), twisting, and kicking Sits with a firm back while propped with pelvic support for up to a half hour Waves and raises arms in anticipation of being picked up and clings when held	Is learning to transfer objects from one hand to the other Reaches for and grasps an object easily Brings her feet to her mouth and sucks on her toes Holds hands together	Awakens at dawn, ready and eager to play Can be alert for one or two hours at a time Resists interruptions in play	Blows "raspberries" (spits bubbles) Babbles to get attention and makes sounds to herself, her toys, or her image in a mirror Shows fear, disgust, or anger by making sounds	Reaches for mommy or daddy and cries if they're out of sight	Still has the tonic neck reflex Doesn't roll over in either direction (front to back or back to side) Seems inconsolable at night Doesn't smile spontaneously Begins babbling but doesn't try to imitate any of your sounds

	Gross Motor	Fine Motor	Cognitive	Language	Social	Warning Signs
Sixth Month	Rolls over in both directions (front to back, back to front) Sits up by herself for a short time, with her head balanced and her hands free Loves to stand (with lots of support) and bounce Rocks back and forth, sometimes crawling backward before moving forward	Uses hands to "rake" small objects Begins to drop things from her high chair, looks for them, and cries for others to pick them up Transfers toys from hand to hand and rotates wrists to turn and manipulate toys Wants to handle all food and utensils	Shows her uniqueness Lets you know how much activity is enough, the amount of sleep she needs, and what foods she prefers Responds to own name Remembers that her primary caregiver exists even when out of sight Shows enjoyment of music by humming, swaying, or bouncing	Babbles by stringing vowels ("ah," "eh," "oh") together, and may start jabbering with consonants Responds to sounds by making sounds Makes sounds to show joy and displeasure	Likes to look at herself in a mirror Knows familiar faces and begins to know if someone is a stranger Likes to play with others, especially parents Watches and plays with a sibling or another child Responds to other people's emotions and often seems happy	Doesn't try to get things that are in reach Has difficulty getting things to mouth Shows no affection for caregivers Cannot sit with help by six months Doesn't make vowel sounds ("ah," "eh," "oh") Doesn't roll over in either direction Doesn't laugh or make squealing sounds
Seventh Month	Moves around—is starting to crawl, scoot, or "army crawl" Supports her whole weight on her legs Sits without support of her hands Bounces when held	Is learning to use thumb and fingers Explores her body Carries a toy much of the time Loves objects that make noise and loves to bang or shake objects to make noise Wants to help with feeding Reaches with one or both hands	Shows tension and irritability before a big developmental step like sitting or crawling Dislikes having a familiar toy removed Resists pressure to do something she doesn't want to do Develops full-color vision and mature distance vision Finds partially hidden object Explores different aspects of a toy	Babbles in a more complex way, says several syllables and uses different ones in the same breath ("ma, mu, da, bah") Begins to respond to "no" Looks from object to parent and back when wanting help (e.g., with a windup toy)	Wants to be included socially Shows increasing dependence on you and fear of separation and strangers Responds to others' expressions of emotion, like tone of voice Smiles, laughs, and has babbling "conversations" with you	Reaches with one hand only Does not actively reach for objects Refuses to cuddle Shows no affection for the person who cares for her Doesn't seem to enjoy being around people Doesn't follow objects with both eyes at one foot to six feet ranges Does not bear some weight on legs

	Gross Motor	Fine Motor	Cognitive	Language	Social	Warning Signs
Eighth Month	Sits well without support Learns to pull herself to sitting and maybe standing positions Empties cabinets, drawers, and bookshelves	Begins to clap hands Pushes away unwanted objects Puts an object into a container and shakes it Picks up a small object with her thumb and two forefingers Holds a bottle to drink	Responds to familiar words Resists bedtimes and naps Repeats sounds or movements she's already made Responds to cues of upcoming events (e.g., blinking before a cup hits the floor or crying when you put on your coat to leave) Solves simple problems (e.g., pushes a button on a toy so it makes a sound)	Babbles with various sounds, inflections, and two-syllable utterances Responds to some requests, like "come here"	Plays interactive games like peekaboo May shout for attention	
Ninth Month	May try to climb or crawl up stairs Stands briefly while you hold her hand Sits up steadily by herself and pivots a quarter of the way around	Finger feeds herself bits of food and drinks from a cup with help Puts her fingers into holes Bangs two objects together	Learns object permanence—that something exists even if she can't see it Looks with interest at pictures in a book Begins to show persistence Enjoys nursery games like pat-a-cake and peekaboo, responds to them, and remembers a game played earlier	Understands and responds to simple commands, like "no-no," "wave," or "clap"	Is at the height of stranger anxiety Performs for familiar audiences and repeats actions if she gets applause or laughs Begins to evaluate and respond to others' moods Prefers watching children to watching adults	

	Gross Motor	Fine Motor	Cognitive	Language	Social	Warning Signs
Tenth Month	Pulls up to stand Stands with little support (for a few moments) Walks while holding on to furniture Lifts her leg to help get dressed May try to climb on furniture (Be careful; she may fall, or the furniture may fall on her.)	Stacks and sorts toys Carries an object in each hand Holds and bites food and may even finger feed herself an entire meal Can Isolate index finger to poke Can drink from a cup	Imitates actions, remembers them, and re- peats them later Remembers where unseen toys are Develops a sense of identity and possession and shows ten- derness toward toys Learns to un- derstand cause and effect ("I cry, Mommy comes")	Lifts up arms to communicate "up" Says "dada" and "mama," though she might not understand them as specific names Understands and obeys some simple commands Imitates non- speech sounds (e.g., coughs, kisses, and tongue clicks)	Becomes self- conscious and sensitive to social approval or disapproval Waves "bye- bye" back	
Eleventh Month	Cruises using furniture Walks holding on to one or two hands Stands without help much of the time Climbs up stairs, but has trouble climbing down (Watch her carefully around the stairs.)	Turns pages while you read Uses two hands at the same time for different functions Experiments with dropping and picking up objects Tries the same activity with each hand or with each side of her body Helps getting dressed more actively Holds a cup and brings a spoon to her mouth Explores containers by lifting their lids and putting objects in	Understands much more than she can say Can look at a picture book on her own	Says "mama" or "dada" for either parent May be able to learn baby sign language Mixes a word into her bab- bling or uses one word to express a whole thought	Uses mealtime games (drop- ping a spoon, pushing food away) to test your reaction May be shy with strangers and play alongside, but not with, another child Resists and tests limits and seeks approval Expresses food preferences	

	Gross Motor	Fine Motor	Cognitive	Language	Social	Warning Signs
Twelfth Month	Takes her first steps; this usually happens right around one year, but it can vary greatly. Stands from a squat, pivots a quarter of the way around, and lowers herself to sit	Helps while getting dressed (pushes hands into sleeves) Begins feeding herself by using a spoon and spills often Begins to use objects correctly (drinking from cup, brushing hair) Uses one hand more than the other Holds a crayon to make marks Pushes toy cars and balls and gives a toy to someone on request	Uses trial and error to solve problems Turns into a very picky eater Becomes resistant, especially at mealtime and naptime	Says an average of two to three words; the range on this is enormous. "Mama" and "Dada" become specific names for parents Points at objects she wants in order to get your attention	Begins "pretend play" by copying you or using objects correctly Has renewed fear of strangers and strange situations Cries when mother or father leaves Shows affection to people and objects	Doesn't crawl; seems to drag one side while she's crawling for a month or more Can't stand with support Doesn't try to find objects you've hidden in front of her Doesn't say any words Doesn't use gestures such as shaking her head "no" and pointing Loses skills she once had

Toys for the First Year

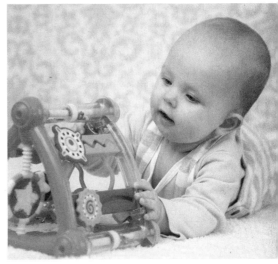

To your baby, everything is a toy—fingers, toes, buttons, strings on clothing, people and pets, household objects, and even pieces of lint. During the first year, she'll play with anything she thinks is a toy to learn about herself and her world. For this reason, make sure her environment is as safe as possible. (See Chapter 4 to learn more about keeping your baby safe.)

Provide new challenges for your baby by offering her toys that aren't too difficult or frustrating and aren't too limited or simple. (See the following pages to help you find toys that fit your baby's developmental abilities.) You don't need to buy lots of expensive toys. Your baby will be perfectly happy playing with homemade toys or with common household objects. For example, you can try one of the following:

- Suspend some colorful pictures from a clothes hanger to make a mobile. (Make sure any strings or cords are secured tightly and out of your baby's reach.)
- Give your baby a set of plastic mixing bowls or containers. She can drop things into and dump things out of them.
- String two or three empty thread spools together to make a simple "clacking" toy.
- Make a homemade book by filling resealable plastic bags with pictures, then sewing the bags together at the seals.
- Make milk carton building blocks: Cut the top off milk cartons and fit two together to form a block.
- Make a glitter bottle: Fill a water bottle using water or oil, then put glitter inside, screw cap back on (tape the cap tightly with duct tape).

Remember, spending one-on-one time reading and singing to your baby, listening to music, and joining her in physical activities such as dancing are far more important than access to a huge array of expensive toys.

Keep in mind the following considerations when buying or making toys for your baby:

Safety

Look for toys that don't have sharp edges or points. Make sure your baby can't break or chew off pieces from them. To make sure your baby won't choke on a toy, choose one that can't fit into a cardboard toilet paper tube (also make sure none of its parts can fit inside). Any cords on toys should be shorter than seven inches, but watch your baby carefully when she's playing with any toy with a cord. Make sure you do not give your baby toys that have any button batteries or magnets.

Check that all parts of the toy are nontoxic. Older toys may have lead paint on them.

Make sure to keep the toys clean by wiping them down or laundering them on a regular basis (especially if your child is getting over an illness).

The Consumer Product Safety Commission (CSPS) is the official federal government agency that issues regularly updated recalls, alerts, and reports on safety of toys and baby equipment. Their website is http://www.cspc.gov.

Durability

Make sure any toy you choose can stand up to any abuse your baby will give it.

Versatility

A good toy stimulates more than one sense. It also has many uses for babies of different ages and developmental levels. For example, some clutch toys are brightly colored, provide faces to look at, are easy to hold, have different textures to touch and mouth, and feature a bell inside to stimulate hearing and encourage shaking or turning.

Toy	Age	Developmental Activity
Pictures	From birth on	Pictures help develop your baby's visual perception (including focus, distance, detail, color, and image recognition). Attach brightly colored or sharply contrasting decals, posters, or other pictures (especially pictures of faces) to your baby's crib, the wall, or a mobile. Make sure the items are out of her reach. At first, your baby can focus on objects only eight to twelve inches. (20.3 to 30.5 cm) away; by four to six months, she can focus on objects across the room.
Books	From birth on	At first, your baby might not show much interest in books, but they play an enormous role in her language development. Read to her as often as you can, at least once a day. Choose books with brightly colored, interesting illustrations. Young babies especially like to look at pictures of faces. Name and describe objects as you point to them on the page. Make animal sounds or tell stories. When she's nine or ten months old, your baby will love handling a book, turning pages back and forth, mouthing it, and dropping it. Make sure the board books you choose are sturdy or expendable—or both.
Mobile	Birth to 2 mos.	A mobile with bright colors and shapes will pique your baby's interest. Choose one that you think will best engage your baby from her perspective. Place it close to her face but out of her reach. Remove the mobile as soon as your baby can move around on her own.
	3 to 4 mos.	At this age, your baby will reach for her mobile as she learns to coordinate her hand movements by grasping at a target. Move the mobile so your baby will also use her feet to try and reach the target. A mobile that makes noise when your baby moves it or kicks the mattress will pique her interest even more. Remember to remove a mobile once your baby can push herself up.

Toy	Age	Developmental Activity
Mirror	2 to 6 mos. and beyond	A mirror helps your baby develop an interest in faces and understand the idea that faces are part of people and that she's an individual. Hang a small, unbreakable mirror on the inside of her crib, above her face as she lies in the crib, or next to the changing table. Your baby will enjoy watching herself and will eventually look into any mirror.
Stuffed animals	2 mos. and beyond	Stuffed animals stimulate lots of activities—an interest in faces (2 mos.), reaching and grasping (3 to 6 mos.), and early manipulation of objects and interest in textures (6 to 18 mos.). A stuffed animal's face may attract your baby, but primarily it's something soft to reach for, grasp, and mouth. Never leave stuffed animals in your baby's crib. If your baby breathes near one too closely while sleeping, she may not get enough oxygen and inhale too much carbon dioxide.
	4 mos. and beyond	Your baby may show affection to one particular stuffed animal. She may see that other children around her often hug, talk to, and pay more attention to a stuffed animal than to other toys. So she may follow suit and become more attached to a stuffed animal than to another toy.
Rattle/ squeak toy	2–4 mos.	Rattles, squeak toys, or anything with bells attached lets your baby watch a moving object and look for the sound source. Move a brightly colored, shiny rattle or squeak toy slowly in front of your baby's eyes. At first, she'll move only her eyes; eventually, she'll move her head, too. Gently shake the rattle or squeak the toy in front of her, then to each side. She'll learn to look for the sound source.
	3–7 mos.	As she gets older, rattles or squeak toys can help your baby develop her ability to reach, grasp, and release. She'll learn to handle, shake, and bang toys. Hold or suspend the toy within your baby's reach. Put it in front of her, then to each side.
Crib gym or exerciser	3–6 mos.	This product provides various objects to look at, pull, push, kick at, and grasp. Set it across the top of your baby's crib or above your baby when she's lying on her back on the floor. Remove a crib gym once your baby can stand.
Ball	3–4 mos.	A brightly colored ball with a noisemaking object inside lets your baby watch a moving object and look and reach for a sound source. Turn or roll the ball slowly in front of your baby.
	4 mos. and beyond	When your baby can roll over, creep, crawl, and finally walk, she'll love a brightly colored, noisemaking ball that she can hold in one hand. She can turn, shake, bang, drop, roll, and chase after it.
Stacking rings	3–6 mos.	The brightly colored stacking pieces are easy to grasp, durable, and smooth. They're perfect objects for your baby to reach for, handle, and mouth.
	9 mos. and beyond	At this age, your baby will learn to control her hand movements so she can stack the objects. At first, your baby will simply stack the objects off the post. When this task no longer challenges her, show her how to put one object on its post and then take it off. Your baby's curiosity and need to imitate will prompt her to stack all the objects on the post.
Small blocks	5–6 mos. and beyond	Blocks are versatile and long-lasting toys. Small, brightly colored blocks are easy to handle and see. Your baby will learn to coordinate her hand movements and pick up and drop blocks into containers. She'll bang blocks together to make noise. Even when she's a preschooler, she can use blocks for building, dramatic play, and learning about size, shape, color, and numbers.
Nesting toys	5–10 mos. and beyond	Nesting toys are objects of the same shape but different sizes that help your baby develop hand coordination and learn that objects exist even when she can't see them. Another way to help your baby learn object permanence is to cover a small toy with a cup, then uncover it. She'll soon play the game herself.

Toy	Age	Developmental Activity
Activity box or cube	6–18 mos.	This toy provides objects that your baby can manipulate, turn, push, poke, or hit. It has various gadgets, like doors to open, balls to spin, and telephone dials to turn.
Pull toys	8 mos. to 2½ yrs.	Pull toys will give your crawling or walking baby a sense of power over objects as well as enjoyment. Many pull toys tip over easily, which will frustrate your baby. Choose a pull toy that's sturdy and stable. Look for one that's brightly colored and makes noise when pulled.
TV, computers, tablets, and cell phones	Birth to 2 yrs.	The American Academy of Pediatrics (AAP) recommends that children younger than age two shouldn't use these devices at all. Your baby's first year is a critical time for growth and development. Her language and social skills will develop far more by talking and interacting with you and others than by watching any program, on any device.
Teething toys	4 mos. and beyond	When babies begin to teethe, they may chew on objects to ease the pain. It's a good idea to purchase a few teething toys to give your baby something safe to mouth. Look for toys that are nontoxic, unbreakable, and big enough that your baby won't swallow them. They may come in animal shapes or look like key rings.

Baby Exercises

Although your baby will likely move her body a lot on her own, the following exercises will work her muscles, test her reflexes, and give you some extra playtime with her, too. Do these exercises on a firm surface and when your baby is alert and content. (Cranky or tired babies will find these exercises annoying, not fun.) Remember to use discretion. Make sure your baby is developmentally ready, for example, when trying the Inchworm.

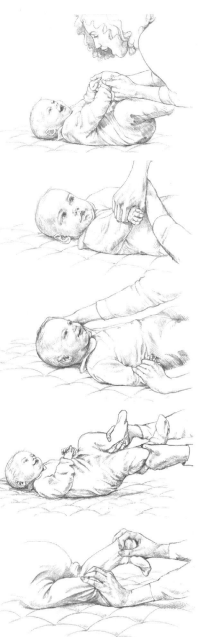

The Grasp: This exercise tests your baby's grasp reflex. Place one index finger in each of your baby's palms. She'll grasp them. Gently pull her hands toward you; she'll pull back on your fingers. (Don't raise her head and shoulders.) If her hands are closed into fists, pat and bounce her hands to open them.

Arm Cross: This exercise relaxes your baby's chest and upper back muscles. Place one thumb in each of your baby's palms. She'll grasp them. Open her arms to the sides and then cross them over her chest. Repeat slowly, gently, and rhythmically.

Arm Raising: This exercise improves the flexibility of your baby's shoulders. Grasp your baby's forearms near the elbows. Raise them above her head, then lower them to the sides. Repeat slowly, gently, and rhythmically. Then alternate arms so one rises while the other lowers.

Leg Bending: This exercise improves the flexibility of your baby's hips. It may also help her pass gas. With your baby on her back, grasp her lower legs and gently bend her knees toward her abdomen and chest. Then gently lower her legs until they're straight. Repeat this exercise several times using both legs, or alternate legs, bending one while straightening the other.

Inchworm: When your baby has some head control, this exercise helps her extend her legs and strengthen her lower back muscles. With your baby on her belly, bend her knees; tuck her legs underneath her body, so her feet are close to her bottom. Press your thumbs against her soles. The pressure will make your baby's legs straighten, which will move her body forward like an inchworm.

Baby Bounce: This exercise relaxes your baby's whole body. Place your baby on her back or belly on a very large, slightly deflated beach ball, a foam pad, a bed, or any soft, bouncy surface. Slowly, gently, and rhythmically press on the area around your baby so she rocks up and down. She'll relax as she feels the movement. Also try patting her rhythmically on her stomach, chest, back, arms, and legs.

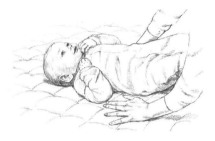

Tummy Time: This exercise encourages proper gross motor development, strengthens neck muscles, and stimulates rolling over. It is also important for normal head-shape growth. Stretch out a clean blanket on the floor, and put your baby on her tummy. At first, keep your face a foot away and talk to your baby, move around a little to encourage her head movement; as she gets stronger, place toys around her, barely within her reach. This should be done a few times a day, for three to five minutes at a time, but you can gradually increase as her neck muscles strengthen. Tummy Time should only be done during awake playtime. Don't leave your baby on her tummy unattended.

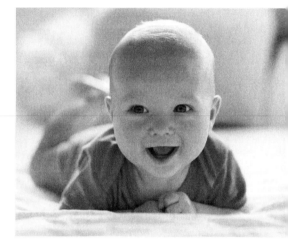

Chapter Six

Medical Care for Your Baby

Making sure your baby is healthy during the first year will help him become a physically and emotionally healthy child and adult. Your baby's well-child checkups are very important. They'll help reduce the number of visits needed for illness or injury. Furthermore, regular checkups will let your baby's health care provider catch any abnormal changes in your baby's growth, development, or behavior. These visits will also give you the opportunity to share with a health care professional what you've experienced, what you've found challenging, and what puzzles you about parenting.

On the following pages, you'll learn more about the well-child checkups and vaccinations recommended for the first year. There's also a section on the development of your child's teeth, a general discussion of how to handle common medical problems, and information on how to treat fever. The chapter concludes with step-by-step treatments for the illnesses and emergencies that your baby may face during his first year.

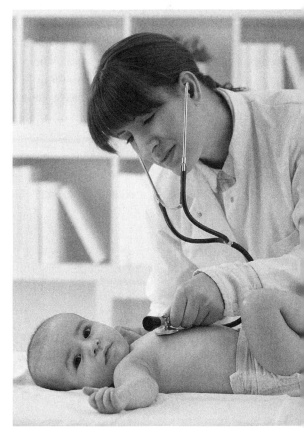

Well-Child Checkups

Because your baby will undergo many developmental changes during the first year, he should have several routine examinations during those months. Your health insurance plan as well as your baby's needs and vaccination schedule will determine when he'll have well-child checkups. (Of course, if he develops health problems that require further attention, his care provider or other health care professionals will see him more frequently.)

With hospitals and birth centers discharging babies earlier than in years past, today's babies generally need a checkup sooner than they did just a decade ago. It is recommended a breastfed baby be checked within forty-eight hours after hospital discharge and all newborns within the first week. He'll have more well-child checkups at the following intervals:

- One month old
- Two months old
- Four months old
- Six months old
- Nine months old
- Twelve months old

At these regular well-child checkups you can expect the care provider to do the following:

- Create a medical record and take a medical history or health profile, including a family history
- Measure your baby's height, weight, and head circumference
- Ask screening questions for vision and hearing
- Ask you questions about iron intake in your baby's diet, lead exposure in your environment, and perform screening blood tests for anemia and lead content in the blood
- Assess developmental and behavioral progress
- Discuss what to expect in your baby's development from one checkup to the next, plus age-related and seasonally relevant topics such as nutrition, sleep, and safety
- Review information on the vaccines recommended at each visit

During the checkup, your baby's care provider will use a stethoscope to listen to your baby's heart and lungs, an otoscope to look into his ears, and a light source (ophthalmoscope and/ or penlight) to check his eyes and mouth. The care provider should also check the abdomen, genitals, hips, and legs.

Well-child checkups are an ideal time to ask questions and share concerns about your baby. If possible, try to use only one or two care providers. This way, you can build a relationship with him or her, and you can discuss your baby's development with someone who's been monitoring it from the beginning.

Vaccinations

Vaccinations are part of most babies' well-child checkups. During the first year, your baby's care provider will recommend that your baby receive vaccinations to protect him against major diseases, including hepatitis B, polio, diphtheria, pertussis (whooping cough), tetanus, hemophilus (Hib) influenzae, rotavirus, influenza, and some strains of pneumococcal disease. A seasonal influenza vaccine will be recommended beginning at six months of age. In total, protection for fourteen diseases before age two will be recommended. Your baby may also be tested for tuberculosis, if there's any risk of exposure to this disease. If you plan on traveling out of the country with your infant, seek additional information about vaccinations recommended for your destination.

A vaccination is a preparation of dead or weakened organisms that's injected into your baby (usually, the upper thigh in infants). A vaccination helps produce immunity to a specific disease by making the body build antibodies to resist the organisms, which protects against future exposure to the disease.

As a parent you may have questions about vaccines. These may focus on a variety of issues:

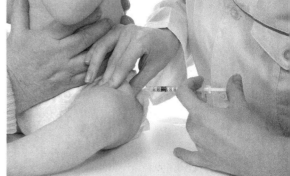

- Are all of these vaccines still necessary now that many of the diseases are so uncommon?

- Do so many vaccines have to be given at one time? Is there a choice of an alternative schedule?

- What about the trauma of the pain of injection? Why can't more vaccines be given by mouth?

- Don't the side effects outweigh the benefits? Is there a relation to autism and vaccines? What about preservatives introducing possibly toxic chemicals into my baby?

The recommended vaccine schedule is updated yearly by the CDC, and disease incidence as well as side effects are monitored very closely. The vaccination of infants and children has resulted in an astounding decrease in serious illnesses and remains a hallmark of maintaining a healthy community both for the infants themselves and for the population at large. The schedule is based on the age that protection is needed as well as when the infant's immunity will respond best. Only a few vaccines induce immunity when given orally, whereas others do not and need to be injected. Many vaccines are now given in combination form so that no more than three injections are needed at one time if the correct schedule is followed. You can discuss with your care provider taking steps that may help reduce the trauma and pain such as breastfeeding during or immediately following the injections and using a calming voice and touch. Vaccines as a cause of autism has been clearly ruled out by several studies, and preservatives are no longer present in significant or potentially harmful amounts.

For more information, please visit these excellent online resources: http://www.cdc .gov, http://www.aap.org, http://www.fda.gov, and http://www.who.int, plus many more resources that are listed in the appendix on pages 217–19.

Though uncommon, some babies have mild reactions to certain vaccines. For example, (usually within twenty-four hours after the vaccination), your baby may become fussy or develop a slight fever or soreness and swelling at the site of the injection. See pages 146–49 to learn how to treat a fever. Take care when moving a sore leg, and apply warm washcloths to the swollen area.

In rare cases, reactions are more severe. True allergic reactions occur in the estimated frequency of about one per million vaccines given. Following are some additional pieces of information that will be helpful to know as you approach bringing your baby in for immunizations:

- Your baby's care provider is required by law to provide you information that explains the potential risks of each vaccine. You should expect to receive a Vaccine Information Statement (VIS) for each of the immunizations your child receives at a well-child visit. Make sure you take this home with you and use it as a reference for education and information on possible side effects.

- Tell your care provider if you, your baby, or another child of yours had a possible significant adverse reaction to a vaccine.

- Ask your care provider whether there are any reasons why your baby shouldn't be vaccinated. For some vaccines, such as influenza, you may be given a checklist to answer about information such as an egg allergy or chronic diseases such as asthma. Some uncommon chronic conditions and infections may serve as contraindications to vaccines.

- If your baby is ill with a fever, the vaccines will likely be postponed. But with most minor illnesses such as the common cold, it is appropriate to proceed with immunizing.

- Report unexpected reactions to your care provider. He or she will report serious reactions to the Vaccine Adverse Event Reporting System (VAERS), a national program for monitoring vaccine safety. You can also contact them yourself at http://www.vaers .hhs.gov/index or 800-822-7967.

- Record the dates and types of vaccinations your baby receives. (The lot numbers of the vaccines will be kept on record at your clinic and sometimes in a state registry format). You'll need the dates and names of the vaccines when you fill out school forms and the like in the future. (Go to http://www.cdc.gov/vaccines/recs/immuniz-records .htm for a printable vaccination form.)

Recommended Vaccination Schedule for the First Year*				
The following schedule may vary slightly among individual clinics and practices as well as for the specific subtype of vaccine given.				
Vaccine	**1st Dose**	**2nd Dose**	**3rd Dose**	**4th Dose**
Hepatitis B**	Birth	1–2 mos.	6–18 mos.	
Rotavirus	2 mos.	4 mos.	6 mos.	
DTaP (diphtheria, tetanus, pertussis)	2 mos.	4 mos.	6 mos.	
Hib (hemophilus influenza type B)	2 mos.	4 mos.	6 mos.	15–18 mos.
Pneumococcal conjugate	2 mos.	4 mos.	6 mos.	12–15 mos.
Inactivated poliovirus	2 mos.	4 mos.	6–18 mos.	
MMR (measles, mumps, rubella)	12 mos.			
Hepatitis A	12 mos.			
Varicella (chicken pox),	12 mos.			
Influenza***	No sooner than 6 mos., during influenza season annually			

* During the second year, your baby will receive additional ("booster") doses of some of the vaccines given in the first year.

** If the mother is a hepatitis B carrier, an additional vaccination should be given.

*** Two doses given at least 4 weeks apart are recommended for children getting their first influenza vaccination. If your baby only gets 1 dose in his first year of vaccination, he should get 2 doses the following year.

If your child falls behind on his immunization, discuss a makeup schedule with your health care provider.

Dental Care

On average, a baby's first tooth appears when he's six to ten months old. Your baby's first tooth, however, could appear any time from birth to eighteen months. The tooth may simply pop through without warning, or your baby may signal its arrival by drooling, fussing, chewing on everything in sight, waking frequently at night, and generally seeming bothered by sore, throbbing gums. Some babies want to nurse or bottle feed more than usual when suffering from teething; others might not. Each baby responds differently to teething. (See pages 207–8 for more on teething.)

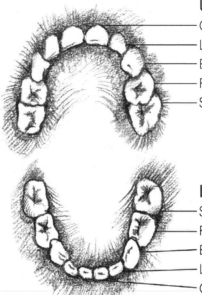

Upper teeth
— Central incisors (8 to 12 months)
— Lateral incisors (9 to 13 months)
— Eyeteeth/cuspids (16 to 22 months)
— First molars (13 to 19 months)
— Second molars (25 to 33 months)

Lower teeth
— Second molars (23 to 31 months)
— First molars (14 to 18 months)
— Eyeteeth/cuspids (17 to 23 months)
— Lateral incisors (10 to 16 months)
— Central incisors (6 to 10 months)

A few more teeth are likely to appear during the first year, and your baby will probably grow a full set of primary (baby) teeth by the time he's two or three. The diagram above shows the average time each primary tooth appears. Don't worry, though, if your baby's teeth come in earlier or later. Girls tend to cut teeth earlier than boys and black babies earlier than white babies.

Start caring for your baby's primary teeth even before they're visible. Healthy baby teeth are essential to the development of your baby's jaw and permanent teeth.

• Feed your baby a nutritious diet. Take him out in the sunshine so his body can produce vitamin D, which strengthens teeth and bones (see page 114). Your care provider may also recommend a vitamin D supplement.

• Fluoride is an important mineral that protects the teeth from acid damage and helps reverse early signs of decay.

Most municipal water sources add fluoride to their water to the concentration of 0.7 parts per million (ppm). Before six months of age a baby only needs 0.1 ppm; from six months until three years of age he only needs 0.3 ppm. Breast milk covers this amount naturally; most formulas do also. To find out how much fluoride is in your drinking water, call your local water department if you drink from a municipal water supply, call the bottling company if you drink bottled water, or ask your local water department about fluoride testing if you drink well water.

Your baby does not need supplemental fluoride during his first six months. It is also not recommended that you mix formula powder or concentrate with water containing fluoride (although it is okay to mix formula with tap water that contains fluoride once in a while). After six months, if your family has a history of weak enamel, or if there are other factors that may weaken his teeth, your care provider may recommend fluoridated water or a fluoride supplement.

- A topical fluoride solution called a varnish may be applied to your baby's teeth at the clinic or in the dental office. It is not recommended to apply over-the-counter topical fluoride rinses at home.

- Fluorosis is a condition that can result from having too much fluoride and presents as very faint white streaks on permanent teeth. It is not painful and does not interfere with the health or function of the teeth.

- Teach your baby how to drink from a cup early on. When your baby's weaned, offer him plenty of foods rich in calcium and vitamin D, like milk, cheese, and yogurt. Calcium is the primary mineral in teeth. Limit the amounts of sticky and sugary foods.

- Don't let your baby use a bottle as a pacifier, and don't put him to bed with a bottle. If he does use a bottle as a pacifier, he may demand several refills of milk or juice, especially at night. This habit encourages decay because it constantly bathes his teeth in sugary liquids (milk contains lactose, a form of sugar). If you decide you must give him a bottle in bed, make sure it contains only water.

- The American Dental Association (ADA) recommends that you start cleaning your baby's teeth as soon as they appear. Gently brush them with a soft, infant toothbrush. Apply a very small amount (about the size of a grain of rice) of toothpaste with fluoride.

- The ADA, American Academy of Pediatric Dentistry (AAPD), and American Academy of Pediatrics (AAP) all suggest that a dentist examine your child within six months after his first tooth comes in and no later than his first birthday. (Local practice may differ—consult with your dentist.) The dentist will check for tooth decay and other problems and show you how to properly clean your baby's teeth. Resource information can be found at http://www.aapd.org.

Fever Guide

Many parents think a fever is their sick baby's number one enemy. They'll battle fever with all the medication and sponge baths they can give their little one. These parents mistakenly believe that a fever in and of itself is a disease that can harm their baby. In reality, a fever is only a symptom of the body's fight against a disease or infection, and the fever in and of itself is generally harmless. When fighting a disease or infection, the body generates excess heat that spreads to the head and limbs, where it radiates off the skin. Almost all infants will have a fever at some point in their early years. What's most important is the search for the cause of the fever.

In general, don't try to bring down a fever that's lower than 100.4°F (38°C) taken rectally, and don't consider a fever alone as a threat to your baby's well-being. You should, however, watch your baby especially closely if he has any fever and he's younger than three months.

Fever Levels

- Rectal temperatures are more accurate than underarm (axillary) temperatures. In infants, the rectal temperature method remains the gold standard. The normal rectal temperature is 99.6°F (37.6°C) (vs. normal oral temperature of 98.6 F), while the normal underarm temperature can range from 96.6°F to 97.6°F (35.9°C to 36.4°C). Further complicating matters, accuracy varies among different thermometers. Remember, nonrectal thermometers don't measure accurate temperatures in babies younger than three months.

- If your baby's underarm temperature is 99°F (37.2°C) or higher, he may have a fever. Use the underarm method to screen for fevers, then take the more accurate rectal method to be sure.

- A high peak temperature for a fever doesn't necessarily mean the disease or infection is comparably severe.

- Unless your baby feels warm to the touch (for example, he feels warmer than your neck) or is acting sick (not eating or sleeping well, increased fussiness, and so on), you don't need to take his temperature.

- A high fever is 104°F (40°C) and higher, no matter which method you use to take a temperature. A fever won't harm a person until it reaches 106°F to 107°F (41.1 to 41.7°C), and fevers of this temperature occur with heatstroke, not common illnesses.

- A person's temperature fluctuates with activity and the time of day. A normal temperature is usually highest in the late afternoon and early evening and lowest between midnight and early morning.

- Teething is not felt to cause a significant elevation of temperature.

- Bundling young infants too warmly and tightly may cause a slight increase in temperature but will not elevate temperature significantly.

- Vaccines may be associated with fever; consult the Vaccine Information Sheet for more specific information following immunizations.

Fever Treatment

- Until your baby is three months old, don't give him any medication until you've called his care provider. Also, never give him aspirin or products that contain aspirin. Aspirin has been linked to Reye's syndrome, a serious condition of progressive vomiting and decreasing consciousness. For more accurate doses that are easier to give to your baby, use infant acetaminophen in liquid form. Infant acetaminophen also comes as rectal suppositories that work well when your baby's vomiting prevents the medicine from staying in his system. Don't use infant ibuprofen until your baby is at least six months old.

- A fever makes a body lose more fluid than usual. To prevent dehydration while he has a fever, encourage your baby to nurse more often or drink more liquids.

- Don't treat a fever with medication until your baby's rectal temperature is higher than 100.4°F (38°C)—and only then if he seems uncomfortable (and only if he is older than three months). Light clothing, extra fluids, and a pleasant, cool room are often better treatments for fevers than medications.

- Don't give your baby cold sponge baths or tub baths, including alcohol baths, to treat a fever, only sponge bathe with tepid water if instructed to do so by your provider.

Recommended Infant Acetaminophen and Ibuprofen Doses for Fever

Note: We are using generic not brand names of antifever medication.

Infant acetaminophen and ibuprofen come in various forms and concentrations. A dropper made by one manufacturer might not give the same amount of medication as another manufacturer's product. Also, most health care providers determine dosages based on a baby's weight, not his age. See the charts on the next page for rough guidelines. If you have questions about dosages, contact your baby's care provider or a pharmacist. Here are more guidelines for giving your baby acetaminophen and ibuprofen:

- Always use the measuring device that comes with the specific product to measure dosages.

- Never give ibuprofen to a baby younger than six months. Do not use ibuprofen if your baby is vomiting constantly or is dehydrated. Don't alternate giving your baby acetaminophen and ibuprofen to treat a fever unless your baby's care provider instructs you to do so.

- Carefully measure and time the doses of acetaminophen or ibuprofen you give your baby. An overdose of fever medication can cause nausea, vomiting, and excessive sweating—it can even be life threatening. If you suspect that your baby has had an overdose, call the national poison control center (800-222-1222) or his care provider immediately.

- If your baby is vomiting and cannot keep an oral medication down, you may want to administer a rectal acetaminophen suppository.

- Never give your baby more than one dose of acetaminophen in any four-hour period or more than five total doses in twenty-four hours. Ibuprofen must not be given any more often than every six hours. The medications should take effect in about twenty to thirty minutes.
- Take your baby's temperature before giving another dose of medication. Taking his temperature can track a rising fever or keep you from giving unnecessary medication.
- Don't awaken your baby to give him medicine or take his temperature—sleep is more important than either.

Recommended Infant Acetaminophen Doses				
Weight	Age	Dosage	Infant Drops	Children's Liquid/Elixir
6–11 lb. (2.7–5 kg)	0–3 mos.	40 mg	1.25 ml	1.25 ml
12–17 lb. (5.5–7.7 kg)	4–11 mos.	80 mg	2.5 ml	½ tsp. (2.5 ml)
18–23 lb. (8.2–10.5 kg)	12–23 mos.	120 mg	3.75 ml	¾ tsp. (3.75 ml)

Recommended Infant Ibuprofen Doses				
Weight	Age	Dosage	Infant Drops	Children's Liquid/Oral Suspension
12–17 lb. (5.5–7.7 kg)	6–11 mos.	50 mg	1.25 ml	½ tsp. (2.5 ml)
18–23 lb. (8.2–10.5 kg)	12–23 mos.	75 mg	1.875 ml	¾ tsp. (3.75 ml)

Contact your baby's care provider in these situations:

- Your baby is younger than three months old and has a rectal temperature of 100.4° F (38°C) or higher; He could have a serious infection, even without other symptoms.
- Your baby is three to six months old with a fever higher than 100.4°F (38.8°C) and he appears ill
- Your baby is any age with a fever higher than 102°F (39.4°C)
- Your baby has a serious disease and has any fever

Note: If your baby has had a convulsion with a fever (febrile convulsion), his care provider may prescribe a slightly different treatment when he has another fever. Febrile convulsions are rare, and a child almost always outgrows them by the time he's six years old. (See pages 203–4.)

How to Take Your Baby's Temperature

For safety's sake, use a digital thermometer and never leave your baby alone while taking his temperature. Glass thermometers can break, and some may contain mercury, a dangerous toxin. The American Academy of Pediatrics (AAP) encourages parents to properly discard mercury thermometers. (See http://www.epa.gov/mercury/spills/index.htm for how to do this.)

Rectal digital thermometers provide the most accurate readings for babies and toddlers. Follow these steps to take your baby's rectal temperature:

1. Clean the tip with rubbing alcohol or soap and water. Rinse with cool water.

2. Put a small amount of lubricant such as petroleum jelly on the tip. Turn on the thermometer.

3. Place your baby on his stomach across your lap or on a firm surface (see illustration). Or put him on his back and hold his ankles in one hand and bend his knees toward his chest.

4. Gently insert the thermometer until the bulb disappears, anywhere from one-quarter to one-half to one inch (6 to 12 millimeters) into the rectum.

5. Hold the thermometer in place loosely with two fingers while keeping your hand cupped around your baby's bottom. When the thermometer beeps, remove it and check the reading. A rectal temperature of 100.4°F (38°C) may mean your baby has a fever.

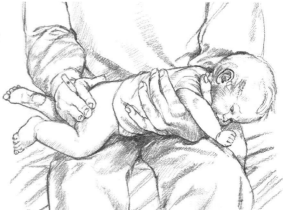

Although less accurate than a rectal temperature, you can use a digital axillary (underarm) thermometer as a first screen. Put the thermometer in your baby's armpit. Bring his arm down and hold it against his body. Wait until the thermometer beeps, and then read it.

You can use an ear thermometer for a baby who is at least three months old. Some parents prefer this thermometer because it's fast and easy to use. You must, however, place it correctly in your baby's ear. Too much earwax may make the reading inaccurate. Gently insert the end of the thermometer in your baby's ear canal, and press the start button. You'll get a reading within seconds.

Don't bother taking your baby's temperature with an oral thermometer; he's simply not mature enough to keep the thermometer in place long enough to get an accurate reading.

Paste strips and pacifier thermometers are less accurate and therefore not recommended.

Handling Common Medical Problems

When your baby is sick or hurt, you want to know quickly what's best to do. The treatments on pages 152–215 will help you care for your baby and tell you when professional help is necessary. These treatments cover common injuries, illnesses, and emergencies that your baby may face during that first year.

The treatments in this section are medically based, but they don't replace professional medical care. An illness's symptoms can vary, and it can affect different children in different ways. Your baby's care provider may need more than one visit to diagnose an illness accurately. He or she may also recommend treatments other than those listed here.

If you have any questions about your baby's health or the best way to handle an illness or injury, contact his care provider. Also, depending on the urgency of the situation, call 911, your health insurance's nurse line, or your baby's care provider if you see any of the following symptoms:

- Any clearly life-threatening injury or accident
- Fever (see pages 146–49)
- Serious diarrhea
- Blood in the urine or stools
- Sudden loss of appetite that lasts four days or longer
- Unusual crying
- Difficulty breathing
- Unusual vomiting
- Off-color appearance, listlessness, or behavioral change
- Convulsions or seizures
- Eye or ear injuries or infections
- Falls or blows to the head that cause unconsciousness (even if brief) or have effects that last longer than fifteen minutes
- Burns with blisters
- Unusual rashes
- Indications of pain (wincing if a spot is touched)
- Suspected poisoning—call national poison control center first (800-222-1222)
- Swallowing a foreign object

Basic Supplies

Here's a list of first-aid and home health care supplies to keep on hand—safely out of your baby's reach:

- Infant acetaminophen or ibuprofen (see pages 147–48 for dosage information)
- Adhesive bandages (assorted sizes)
- Adhesive tape one-half to one inch wide
- Cool-mist humidifier or vaporizer
- Cotton balls
- Cotton safety swabs (designed for children)
- Diaper rash cream or ointment
- Baby nail clippers
- Heating pad
- Hot-water bottle
- Nasal aspirator (bulb syringe)
- Rubbing alcohol
- Sunblock (at least SPF 15 and PABA-free)
- Digital thermometer (For a newborn, use a rectal or underarm thermometer. An ear thermometer is appropriate after your baby is three months old.)
- Tweezers

Symptoms Index

If you're perplexed by what illness your baby may have, look up the symptoms you've noticed in this index. See what other symptoms match (or don't match) your baby's. Then make an educated guess about what illness your child has. Don't use this index to play doctor, and don't assume that every baby with bronchiolitis, for example, has every symptom listed under that entry. Work closely with your baby's care provider if you have any doubts about your baby's symptoms.

Acne (Newborn)

Description

Newborn acne is a condition in which a newborn's skin breaks out in pimples. Up to 20 percent of babies may get acne. The cause is not fully understood.

What You Need to Know

- Newborn acne is common and usually clears up on its own. It often appears when a baby is about three weeks old and disappears or improves significantly without treatment, usually in days or weeks but almost always by four months. Another type of acne, called infantile acne, can appear later, be more severe, and is almost always gone by one year of age.
- Oily areas produce the most pimples: around the nose, on the cheeks or back, or near the scalp.
- If your baby has small red bumps in the folds of his skin, he probably has heat rash, not acne. See page 190 for more on heat rash.

Supplies

Washcloth, soap, and water

Symptoms

- Blackheads (pimples with dark centers)
- Whiteheads (pimples with white centers)

Get Professional Help If:

Your baby's skin seems especially dry, irritated, weepy, or possibly infected

What to Check

- Does your baby's acne seem to be spreading rapidly and causing discomfort?

Treatment

- Wash the affected skin daily and gently with soap on a wet washcloth, then pat the area dry. The clogged pores should open and heal by themselves without further treatment.
- Make sure your baby sleeps on clean sheets that are washed with gentle detergents.
- Don't use over-the-counter acne medication or creams, oils, or lotions. In rare, severe cases, your baby's care provider may prescribe a medication.

Anaphylaxis

Description

Anaphylaxis (also called anaphylactic shock) is a sudden, severe, potentially fatal, allergic reaction to insect bites or to certain foods (like nuts), materials (like latex), and medications (like penicillin). Though rare, true anaphylaxis is always an emergency.

What You Need to Know

- Symptoms may begin in as little as five minutes to two hours after exposure to the allergen, but life-threatening reactions may progress over hours.
- Some people have a reaction, and the symptoms go away only to return two to three hours later. Often the symptoms occur in the respiratory tract and take the person by surprise.
- Anyone with a history of anaphylactic reactions is at risk for another severe reaction. Those with food allergies and asthma may be at increased risk for having a life-threatening anaphylactic reaction.

Supplies

- Epinephrine auto-injector device; antihistamines, if prescribed by a medical professional

Symptoms

- Hives (raised red patches of skin), and swelling of the throat, tongue, neck, or face

- Puffiness of the face, eyelids, ears, mouth, hands and feet (angioedema)
- Wheezing or severe breathing problems
- Rapid pulse and decreased blood pressure
- Sweating
- Dizziness, fainting, loss of consciousness
- Nausea, vomiting, abdominal cramps, diarrhea
- Extremely pale skin or skin turning blue

Get Professional Help If:

Your baby has difficulty breathing, becomes unconscious, or has a combination of the above symptoms

What to Check

- If your baby has had previous reactions, learn to recognize the symptoms and call for professional help or follow prescribed treatment.

Treatment

- The best treatment is to avoid the allergens that cause reactions.
- If your baby is at risk for anaphylaxis, his care provider should prescribe an epinephrine auto-injector device for emergency use and train you to use it. During an emergency, administer the prescribed medicine and call 911.
- Your baby may need to wear a medical identification bracelet.

Bites and Stings
(Insect, Animal, or Human Bites)

Description

Bites or stings can make an impression in or break the skin. Insects including mosquitoes, flies, fleas, bedbugs, fire ants, ticks, chiggers, and spiders may spread disease such as encephalitis, malaria, and Lyme's disease via their bites. Bees, wasps, and hornets sting using the back parts of their bodies. They do not carry disease but their stings can cause an allergic reaction that can be serious and even cause anaphylaxis.

What You Need to Know

- Don't use insect repellents that contain DEET (diethyltoluamide) on babies younger than two months. Instead, dress your baby in long sleeves and pants to cover as much of his skin as possible. If you use a DEET repellent on your child, choose one that contains no more than 30 percent DEET, don't apply it more than once a day, apply to clothes and sparingly on skin, and don't apply it to your child's hands or around his nose, eyes, or mouth. Don't apply it on cuts, wounds, or irritated skin. Wash treated skin and clothing after returning indoors. Avoid spraying DEET in enclosed areas or near food. If you want to use a DEET-free insect repellent, choose those containing eucalyptus oil or soybean oil; another option to ask your care provider about is picaridin. Unfortunately, all of these repellants offer protection against the common biting insects but no protection against stinging insects (bees, hornets, and wasps).

- Most animal bites come from family or neighborhood pets. Dogs, cats, and snakes are the most common biting animals. Some infants experience emotional trauma from being bitten. Always supervise your baby when he's in a room with animals. Watch for any aggressive or defensive behaviors.

- Human bites become infected more often than animal bites.

- Deep bite wounds may require stitches, and stitches increase the chances of infection.

- Insect bites usually cause only mild, local reactions; in rare cases, however, they can cause more severe allergic reactions, such as anaphylaxis. (See page 153.)

- Scented soaps attract insects.

Supplies

Soap and water, washcloth, a bee-sting kit for allergic infants, calamine lotion, baby nail clippers

Symptoms

Signs of an infected wound include the following:

- Pus or drainage coming from the bite

- Swelling, tenderness, and warmth around the bite

- Red streaks spreading from the affected area

- Swollen glands in the area of the bite

Get Professional Help If:

- Your baby's been bitten on the face, hands, feet, or genital area.
- The bite wound is large.
- A deep puncture wound has occurred, especially if it involves bone, tendons, or joints.
- There's any concern that a rabies-infected animal bit your baby. If this is the case, try to have the animal captured and checked for rabies. Wild animals most likely to transmit rabies are bats, skunks, raccoons, coyotes, and foxes. Domestic cats and dogs need to have been vaccinated for rabies to be considered safe from transmission.
- The wound appears infected or extremely swollen, or red streaks appear to spread out from the bite.
- Your baby has trouble breathing after an insect bite. (See page 153.)
- His itching is severe or hives appear.

What to Check

- Keep an eye on your baby after a bite, and watch for signs of infection or trouble breathing.
- Make sure vaccinations for tetanus and hepatitis B are up to date.

Treatment

- To stop bleeding, apply firm pressure to the wound for up to five minutes.
- Wash the wound with soap and water.
- Use calamine or other anti-itch lotions to soothe insect bites.
- For a bee or wasp sting, apply pressure to the wound with a cold, wet washcloth to reduce swelling. If you can see the stinger, try to remove it by scraping your fingernail gently across the wound.
- If a tick is present, try to remove it using tweezers; grasp the tick as close to your baby's skin as possible, and pull straight out. If any part of the tick is still in his skin, remove those parts with clean tweezers. Wash the affected area with soap and water.
- Trim your baby's nails to prevent scratching. (See page 42.)
- To prevent bites, avoid dressing your baby in bright colors and cover as much of his skin as possible with clothing. Mosquito netting may be helpful as well. Avoid areas and times of day when insects are most plentiful. Keep door and window screens in good repair.

Breathing Emergency/Cardiac Arrest

Description

If your baby's breathing or heartbeat stops, it's a life-threatening situation. In infants, most cardiac arrests are caused by lack of oxygen such as from respiratory failure, drowning, or choking. In 2010, the American Heart Association updated its guidelines to recommend everyone begin cardiopulmonary resuscitation (CPR) with chest compressions to keep blood circulating to the brain. Remember the new acronym, C-A-B (circulation, airway, breathing).

What You Need to Know

- Time is critical. Act quickly while someone else calls for help.
- If your baby isn't breathing due to choking and he's still conscious but unable to vocalize, follow the procedures on pages 160–61 to try to dislodge the object, then begin CPR if needed (see page 157).
- If your baby isn't breathing due to electric shock, don't touch him directly if he's still touching the electrical source. Turn off the electric current, remove the fuse (or trip the circuit breaker), or stand on a nonconducting mat, like a rubber doormat, and push him away from the source with a nonconducting object, like a dry wood board. Never use a wet or metal object.
- If your baby isn't breathing due to anaphylaxis (see page 153), administer any prescribed medication and call 911.
- If you don't know why your baby isn't breathing and you're trained in CPR, use the techniques on page 157. If you're not trained, you should still do continuous chest compressions (about one hundred a minute, one and a half inches down the chest) to keep blood flowing to the brain and body.
- Don't tilt your baby's head if you suspect a head or neck injury. Many falls result in a head or neck injury. Instead, a trained professional should use the jaw-thrust technique. If no professional is with you and you're losing time, then you should perform the head-tilt/chin-lift method (see step 4, page 157), as getting oxygen to the brain takes priority.

Supplies

None

Get Professional Help If:

Your baby's heartbeat or breathing stops and he's unconscious. Have someone else call 911 and follow the steps for CPR while waiting for help. If you're alone, begin CPR for at least two minutes or five cycles before you call 911. Don't stop CPR for longer than a minute. Continue until help arrives or your baby has a pulse and is breathing on his own.

Treatment

If your baby is choking, see pages 160–61 for procedures. Otherwise, see the following instructions for infant CPR. CPR for babies younger than one year differs from the technique used for older children. A CPR course prepares you best for this emergency, but you should try chest compressions even if you're untrained.

CPR Step-by-Step

Step 1: Gently touch your baby to see whether he's unconscious. If conscious, he'll respond and breathe. (If he responds but does not breathe, he may be choking. See pages 160–61 for procedures.) Don't take more than ten seconds to try to determine if he's breathing, and don't check for a pulse unless you are a trained health professional. If you don't get a response, lay him on his back and begin CPR, starting with compressions.

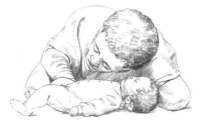

Step 2: Place two fingers on the breastbone at or just below an imaginary line connecting the nipples. Gently press your fingers about one and a half inches into the chest (or at least one-third of the thickness of the chest). Let the chest come all the way up after a compression. Do this thirty times at a rate of about two compressions per second, or at least one hundred compressions per minute. If you're not trained in CPR, continue to do compressions until help arrives. If you are trained, continue to step 3.

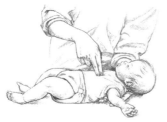

Step 3: After thirty compressions, clear the airway. Tilt your baby's head by lifting his chin with one hand and pushing down on his forehead with the other. (If you suspect a head or neck injury, and a trained professional is with you, he or she should do the jaw-thrust technique instead. If a trained professional is not present, then use the head-tilt/chin-lift method (step 4), since getting oxygen to the brain takes priority.) Quickly (no more than ten seconds) check for breathing. Listen for breaths and look for chest movement.

Step 4: With your baby's head still tilted, cover his entire mouth and nose with your mouth and gently blow until you see his chest rise. Let air escape as his chest goes down. Give two breaths over about two seconds. If no air goes in, adjust his head and try one more time.

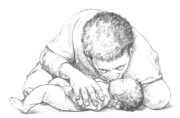

Step 5: Go back to compressions. Continue to alternate thirty compressions with two rescue breaths until help arrives. Do not check for a pulse unless you are a trained health professional, as this may delay important resuscitation. If two people are available to do CPR, the rate of compression to rescue breaths can be fifteen to two.

Note: According to the American Academy of Pediatrics (AAP), it is now acceptable to use an AED (automated external defibrillator) on infants less than one year of age in cardiac arrest (no pulse). Pediatric pads are recommended, but adult pads can be used if necessary. Have someone bring an AED if one is available and follow the instructions to use it.

Bronchiolitis and Asthma
(Typical Causes of Wheezing in Babies)

Description

Bronchiolitis is an acute inflammation and swelling of the smallest air passages (bronchioles) that is common in infants less than two years and usually caused by a viral infection, most often respiratory syncytial virus (RSV). Asthma refers to a chronic condition that predisposes one to wheezing; it can be triggered by things like an infection or an allergy.

What You Need to Know

- Bronchiolitis occurs mostly in babies. Bronchitis is the infection of larger airways, and it's rare in babies.
- Bronchiolitis has many of the same symptoms as pneumonia.
- It usually lasts several days or even weeks but will eventually disappear on its own.
- RSV infections are most common between October and March.
- Ear infections can accompany bronchiolitis.
- Bronchiolitis may put some children at risk for developing asthma.
- The virus that causes bronchiolitis is highly contagious. Careful hand washing and use of alcohol-based hand sanitizers help prevent spread.
- Some high-risk infants qualify to receive a preventive antibodies-based series of injections during the winter months to help prevent getting RSV. Speak with your care provider if you think your infant may qualify.

Supplies

Thermometer, prescribed medication, clear liquids, cool-mist humidifier or nebulizers

Symptoms

- Runny nose
- Rapid, shallow breathing up to sixty to eighty times per minute
- Labored breathing:
  - Periods of apnea (breathing may stop temporarily for more than ten seconds); this is more likely to happen in premature and young infants.
  - Nostrils widen and move more often.
  - Muscles between the ribs move in and out (increased work to breathe).
  - Grunting sounds with exhalation
  - Wheezing (a high-pitched noise, especially when exhaling)
- Fever (See pages 146–49.)
- Cough, often raspy
- Loss of appetite

Get Professional Help If:

- Your baby has the above symptoms, especially if his breathing is rapid or labored.
- His lips, skin, or fingertips appear bluish, or breathing seems to tire him.
- He refuses fluids because he is working too hard to breathe. Dehydration may occur.
- He has another medical condition, like heart, lung, neurologic, or immune

disease, or prematurity, while having bronchiolitis symptoms.

- Your baby is less than twelve weeks of age and develops bronchiolitis.

What to Check

- Note temperature daily (see page 149).
- Monitor symptoms.

Treatment

Follow the treatment recommended by your baby's care provider. It may include the following:

- Avoid any smoke exposure.
- Frequent breast milk, formula, or clear liquids
- Humidify the air.
- Use a nasal aspirator with saline drops.
- Some babies require supplemental oxygen in the hospital for supportive treatment.

Choking
(Foreign-Body Aspiration)

Description

This is a life-threatening obstruction of the airway caused by an object or food.

What You Need to Know

- Choking signals include bluish lips, nails, and skin; the inability to vocalize, breathe, or cry; high-pitched cries; and ineffective coughs.

- If your baby can still vocalize, cry, cough, breathe, sputter, or move air at all, don't interfere with him or call for help. His normal reflexes will best clear and open his airway. Let him cough to try to remove the object. If this doesn't work and you can see the object, you can try to sweep it out, but be careful not to push it farther into his mouth.

- If your baby has stopped breathing, start treatment first, then call for help. Or have someone else get help while you begin treatment.

Supplies

None

Get Professional Help If:

Your baby can't vocalize, cry, cough, or breathe, and he's turned blue or he is unconscious. Have someone call 911 for help while you begin emergency procedures.

Treatment

Note: The following instructions are for babies younger than age one. Techniques for older children are different.

If your child is conscious but unable to vocalize or cry, follow these steps. After performing these procedures for one minute, call 911 if your baby's not breathing and the object hasn't been dislodged. If your baby becomes unconscious, begin infant CPR. See page 157.

Step 1: Place your baby facedown on your forearm, keeping his head lower than his body. Support his jaw and chest with your hand. Rest the arm holding him on your thigh, pressing the upper arm against your body for further support. Use the heel of your free hand to give five quick blows (backslaps) between his shoulder blades.

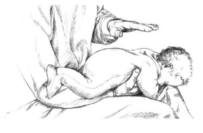

Step 2: If the object doesn't dislodge, place your free arm along his spine and cradle his head in your hand. Then carefully turn your arm so it rests on your thigh and your baby is face-up (his head still lower than his body). Use two fingers to give five quick thrusts (one inch deep) into the breastbone between the nipples and one finger-width below them.

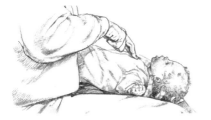

Step 3: Repeat steps 1 and 2 until the object is dislodged (call 911 after one minute or your baby becomes unconscious. If he becomes unconscious, begin CPR. See page 157.

If your baby coughs up the object and starts to breathe, still call 911. If you can see the object, but your baby has not coughed it out, you can try to sweep it out, but be careful not to push it farther into the mouth.

Cold and Cough
(Upper Respiratory Infection, Common Cold)

Description

A cold is a common, contagious viral infection of the nasal and throat membranes, sometimes also affecting the ears and chest. Colds are almost always mild and get better on their own. A cough is a reflex response to infection or irritation in the respiratory system.

What You Need to Know

- Newborns and young babies often sneeze mucus that's left over from birth. This is not a signal of a cold.
- Many babies have six to eight colds per year in the first few years, most frequently between September and April.
- Colds are most contagious in the first two to four days; symptoms usually subside by ten to fourteen days without treatment. Colds spread most commonly through coughing, sneezing, and hand contact.
- Antibiotics don't cure colds (because colds are caused by viruses, not bacteria) and may worsen them or upset a baby's stomach.
- Ear infections (viral and bacterial) are the most common complication of colds. Pneumonia, sinus infection, and asthma can also be complications.
- Coughs can be caused by things other than infections, including swallowing a foreign object, allergies, and asthma.
- Coughing itself is a good thing as it helps clear out the respiratory system.
- A forceful cough may cause vomiting.

Supplies

Thermometer, liquids, nasal aspirator, infant acetaminophen or ibuprofen (babies younger than six months should not take ibuprofen; see pages 147-48 for dosage information), and saline drops (available over the counter)

Symptoms

- Congested, runny nose, with thin and clear mucus early on but often thick and colored as the cold progresses
- Red, watery eyes
- Sneezing
- Hoarseness
- Difficulty breathing
- Listlessness or irritability
- Decreased appetite
- Fever (See pages 146-49.)
- Sore throat or difficulty swallowing
- Mild swelling of the lymph nodes

Get Professional Help If:

- His breathing seems labored or rapid.
- His lips or fingernails are bluish.
- He becomes particularly irritable or listless.
- He seems to have pain or is tugging at one or both ears.
- He has a fever of 100.4°F (38°C) or higher and is less than three months. (See pages 146-49.)
- He is refusing feedings.

What to Check

- Take your baby's temperature if he seems warm or sick. (See page 149.)
- Note whether the cough is worse during the day, night, or both.

Treatment

- Make sure your baby remains well hydrated.
- If your baby's younger than six months old, using a nasal aspirator may help to gently clear mucus from his nose before feedings and naps. If this procedure causes discomfort or irritation, try using normal saline drops. You may also combine both of these techniques. Place your baby on his back, insert a couple of drops of saline into each nostril, then wait for a few minutes for the mucus to soften. Next, take your nasal aspirator (if you are using a bulb syringe, squeeze it to remove most of the air); gently insert the small open tip into your baby's nostril and move it around in the nostril to draw out the mucus (if you are using a bulb syringe, slowly release the bulb to suck in mucus).

- Talk to your baby's care provider about giving your baby infant acetaminophen or ibuprofen or any over-the-counter medications. Ibuprofen should not be used before six months of age and acetaminophen for colds is not recommended for infants less than three months. (Over-the-counter cold medications can thicken mucus and have other side effects.)
- A cool-mist humidifier may help thin the mucus. Make sure you clean the humidifier according to the manufacturer's instructions.
- Avoid any exposure to smoke.
- It is not recommended to use topical rubs such as those with menthol products or herbal, zinc, or vitamin C preparations.
- Frequent hand washing and cough hygiene for caregivers may help prevent the spread of the common cold.

Colic

Description

Prolonged periods of daily intense and excessive crying in babies is called colic. It is one of the most distressing problems of infancy. One definition of colic is "a baby who cries more than three hours a day, more than three days a week, and is less than three months old." Although there isn't a fully understood medical explanation, a colicky baby may have an immature nervous system, causing him to be sensitive to stimulation and unable to be consoled. A colicky baby's cry is often louder, more intense, and higher pitched than a typical cry. The belly can be hard, the arms stiffened, the fists clenched, and the back arched.

What You Need to Know

- One in five babies gets colic, usually beginning between the ages of two and four weeks and lasting about three months. Sixty percent of babies resolve their colic by three months and 90 percent by four months.
- A baby with colic will grow and show normal development.
- Because there's no definite or obvious reason for the crying—which may continue for hours—colic can frustrate parents.
- Some evidence suggests that a nursing mother's consumption of cow's milk or other potentially irritating foods like eggs, nuts, and wheat can cause some cases of colic. You can try eliminating these foods from your diet one at a time and checking your baby's response.

- Babies who are fed cow's milk–based formula may become less colicky if offered a hydrolyzed-protein formula. You should be able to tell in a few days to one week if this makes a difference.
- Almost all babies are fussy in the evening during the first few months; this fussy period is not colic.
- Some babies are fussy because of gastroesophageal reflux disease (see pages 184–85).
- It is a myth that babies can cry to manipulate parents at this age, or that babies can be spoiled if you hold them too much.

Supplies

Thermometer, pacifier, hot-water bottle or heating pad, bottles and nipples that prevent swallowing air

Symptoms

- Inconsolable crying that persists around the clock but is usually worse in the early evening
- Acting hungry, but then crying halfway through feeding
- Drawing up the legs to the body; clenching fists

Get Professional Help If:

- You suspect colic but want reassurance that there's no other medical problem.
- Your baby cries persistently for more than two to four hours.
- There is a fever (see pages 146–49), runny nose, cough, vomiting, or other signs of illness.

- Symptoms don't significantly improve by the time your baby's four months old.
- You need support to help you cope.

What to Check

- Possible causes of discomfort, like illness, diaper rash, or constipation (hard stools)
- If you are formula feeding, make sure you prepare the formula properly. Also make sure the formula flows from the nipple at about one drop per second.

Treatment

- There's no surefire treatment, so try various methods to soothe your baby. It's possible no method will work. Be patient as you try these methods:
  - Cuddling, swaddling (see pages 25–26), rocking, walking your baby, keeping him upright by carrying him or placing him in a sling or front carrier
  - Taking him on a trip in a car
  - Using a pacifier or "white noise," such as a recorded heartbeat or sounds of nature, vacuum cleaner, hairdryer, washing machine, or clothes dryer (Don't place your baby in any type of carrier on top of a dryer.)
  - Laying him facedown across your knees and rubbing his back
  - Burping him frequently
  - Applying mild heat to his abdomen, rubbing his belly
  - Giving him a warm bath
- Don't overstimulate your baby by jiggling or moving him too much.

- No matter how distraught you're feeling, *never* shake your baby. This can cause blindness, brain damage, or death. If you are feeling distraught and need someone to talk to, call the twenty-four-hour hotline at 800-4-A-CHILD (800-422-4253).
- If you're nursing your baby, eliminate cow's milk from your diet for two weeks to see whether that reduces your baby's symptoms. A diet free of eggs, nuts, and wheat may help. If you are bottle feeding, a one-week trial of a hydrolyzed-protein formula may help.
- Don't overfeed your baby as this may make him more uncomfortable. You shouldn't need to feed him more often than every two hours (from the start of one feeding to the start of the next).
- It's okay to take a ten- to fifteen-minute break from trying to console your baby if nothing seems to be working. Place him in a safe position in a safe place.
- Remember: Colic is temporary and will disappear when your baby's older (usually when he's around three months old).
- Arrange for someone else to care for your baby, even if only for a few hours. It's critical that you get a break every now and then.
- Discuss your frustration with others. Having a colicky baby is not caused by bad or poor parenting. Support from others will help you handle the stress and frustration that can come from having a baby with colic.

Constipation

Description
Your baby has constipation if he has hard (possibly large and dry or small and pebbly) bowel movements that are difficult to pass.

What You Need to Know
- Constipation is often overdiagnosed. Diet or illness may cause hard bowel movements; more rarely, a congenital defect of the nerve cells of the anus (Hirschsprung's disease) causes them. Breastfed babies are rarely constipated.
- It's normal for babies to strain and turn quite red while passing a normal bowel movement. This alone does not mean a baby is constipated.
- Constipation tendency may run in families, which can put an individual baby at higher risk.
- Constipation refers more to stool consistency than frequency. Babies differ greatly in their bowel habits. After one to two months of exclusive nursing, breastfed babies may have very infrequent bowel movements.
- Iron-containing formulas do not cause constipation, since the amount of iron in them is small.
- When you start your baby on solid foods, his stools will often change. Rice cereal and bananas tend to cause constipation, so balance these foods with high-fiber ones, like fiber-containing cereal (whole wheat, barley), peas, and prunes. The recommended daily amount of fiber is 5 grams for this age.
- A small tear in the anus called an anal fissure may make bowel movements painful and even bloody. Avoid too vigorous wiping at diaper change time to prevent aggravating these.

Supplies
Fruits, juices such as prune, pear, and apple, water

Symptoms
- Hard pellet-like stools
- Stools that have blood in or on them
- Painful bowel movements
- Abdominal pain relieved after having a bowel movement
- Arching of the back, tightening of the buttocks, crying
- More frequent spitting up

Get Professional Help If:
- Your baby's bowel movements seem painful, with the pain lessening afterward.
- His stools are bloody either on the inside or outside.
- His stools are pellet-like, firm, and dry.
- He's constipated frequently.
- His constipation doesn't improve with home treatment.

What to Check
Is your baby drinking fewer fluids than usual or eating more solid foods that cause constipation?

Treatment

- Try giving your baby (older than one month) one ounce per month of age of undiluted prune, apple, or pear juice. For example, give three ounces to a three-month-old. Give four to eight ounces to four- to eight-month-olds and eight to twelve ounces to eight- to twelve-month-olds. You may need to adjust the amounts for more effectiveness.

- If your baby's eating solid foods, consider giving him more high-fiber solids, like peas, beans, broccoli, apricots, plums and prunes, sweet potatoes, peaches, pears, and spinach.

- Give your baby more water.

- If giving your baby more water and high-fiber foods does not work, then try adding dark corn syrup to expressed milk or formula as another remedy. A mixture of one teaspoon per four ounces of milk or formula, not to exceed a total of one to two tablespoons a day.

- Before giving your baby laxatives, enemas, suppositories, or mineral oil, first call your baby's care provider. Don't try to stimulate a bowel movement with a rectal thermometer unless the care provider has instructed you to do so.

Cradle Cap
(Seborrheic Dermatitis, Dandruff)

Description

Cradle cap is a noncontagious skin and/or scalp condition recognized by oily, yellowish scales or crusted patches.

What You Need to Know

- Cradle cap is most common in babies (it is reported in up to 10 percent of infants less than one month old) but occurs in children as old as six years.
- It usually appears on the scalp but may appear as reddish scales wherever there's a concentration of oil-producing glands (forehead, eyebrows, behind the ears, upper chest, back, or groin).
- It can be a recurring condition but will often improve by itself during the first month.
- It isn't harmful, isn't related to poor hygiene, and will eventually disappear on its own. It doesn't itch or cause discomfort.
- It can be treated, but treatment isn't necessary.

Supplies

Washcloth, soap and water, baby shampoo, petroleum jelly, fine-tooth comb or brush, baby oil, towel

Symptoms

- Yellowish scales
- Crusty skin patches surrounded by slight redness

Get Professional Help If:

- The condition persists after several weeks of home treatment.
- Your baby's skin becomes infected.

What to Check

Watch for signs of skin infection.

Treatment

- Use a washcloth, soap, and water to wash the affected areas daily. For the scalp, shampoo the hair frequently (daily if necessary) with a mild, non-medicated baby shampoo.
- Remove scales with a fine-tooth comb, soft brush, or soft toothbrush.
- For stubborn cases, try rubbing a little baby oil into the affected areas, and cover with a warm towel for fifteen minutes. Then shampoo, gently massage the scalp, and work the scales loose with a comb, and rinse.
- If nothing else works, talk with your baby's care provider about using a medicated shampoo that helps dissolve the scales or a cortisone cream or lotion.

Crossed Eyes
(Strabismus)

Description

Crossed eyes, or strabismus, is the inward or outward turning of one or both eyes rather than parallel eye motion or position. It's caused by an imbalance of the muscles that control eye movement, resulting in an inability to focus on the same point at the same time.

What You Need to Know

*   Many newborns have eyes that periodically wander. The condition usually improves markedly by the time a baby is two to three months old.

*   Premature babies are at a higher risk for developing crossed eyes than full-term babies.

*   Your baby's eyes will be checked at routine well-child care visits—let your care provider know if your baby is not making regular eye contact or is not tracking objects by three months of age.

Supplies

None

Symptoms

For a baby older than two to three months:

*   One or both eyes crossing most or all of the time

*   Eyes not tracking together

Get Professional Help If:

Your baby's eyes seem crossed, appear to wander, or don't seem to track together after the first few months. Even intermittent crossed eyes after age three months need evaluation. If you have any concerns, see an ophthalmologist or eye specialist recommended by your baby's care provider. If your baby's condition is serious, it must be treated to prevent vision problems.

What to Check

If the bridge of your baby's nose is flat and he has skin folds on the insides of his eyes, it may seem as though he has crossed eyes. He doesn't; this is a condition called pseudostrabismus. No treatment is necessary, and the appearance will improve over time.

Treatment

*   There aren't any home remedies. If you suspect your baby has crossed eyes, have your baby's care provider recommend an eye specialist to evaluate him.

*   Medical treatment may involve eye drops, wearing a patch over one eye, wearing prescription glasses, or undergoing surgery.

Croup

Description

Croup is a barking cough and/or labored breathing caused by inflammation and swelling of the windpipe (trachea) and voice box (larynx). The cough is often described as sounding like a seal bark, dog bark, or frog croak.

What You Need to Know

- A croup attack may be preceded by a fever and nasal stuffiness but often appears suddenly (usually at night), for no apparent reason. It requires immediate home treatment.

- Children between the ages of three months and three years are the most susceptible because their airways are narrow.

- If the attack is severe and doesn't respond to home treatment, it may require medical treatment.

- A virus almost always causes croup, but allergies may be a factor as well. Bacterial causes have decreased thanks to protection from vaccines.

- Croup most frequently appears in the late fall and winter.

- If your child has recurrent bouts of croup, discuss further treatment with his care provider.

Supplies

Thermometer, cool-mist humidifier or vaporizer, infant acetaminophen or ibuprofen (babies younger than six months should not take ibuprofen; see pages 147–48 for dosage information), liquids

Symptoms

- A hacking cough
- Difficulty breathing
- Fever (See pages 146–49.)
- Hoarseness
- Noisy, high-pitched breathing, especially when baby is active or upset

Get Professional Help If:

- Symptoms rapidly worsen, and home treatment doesn't help enough to let your baby fall asleep.

- Your baby's fever is higher than 103°F (39.4°C) or, if less than three months, 100.4°F (38°C).

- He turns blue, drools, or struggles to breathe.

- He can't speak or make verbal noises.

- He is very upset, very sleepy, or seems to be unresponsive.

- Croup becomes a recurrent or persistent issue for your baby.

What to Check

Don't leave your baby alone during an attack. Because an attack may occur several nights in a row, watch him closely for three nights.

Treatment

- Try to keep your baby as calm as possible by using your usual soothing techniques.

- Although you can treat most cases at home, contact your baby's care provider if your baby's breathing doesn't improve.

- Take your baby into the bathroom, close the door, and run a hot shower to generate steam while you sit near the shower with your baby for fifteen to twenty minutes.

- Instead of steam or if steam doesn't help, take your baby into cool, moist outside air for twenty minutes. If there's still no improvement, call 911 or his care provider immediately.

- If the care provider prescribes a home treatment, put a cool-mist humidifier or vaporizer in the room, and give him liquids and infant acetaminophen or ibuprofen. (See pages 147–48 for dosage information.)

- Make sure your baby remains well hydrated.

- Your care provider may prescribe oral or injectable steroids to help decrease the inflammation and swelling.

- Don't give your baby cough syrup.

- Avoid any exposure to smoke.

- Don't try to open your baby's airway by putting your finger in his mouth. The swollen tissue causing the obstruction can't be cleared away.

Dehydration

Description

Dehydration means there's an insufficient amount of fluid in the body. It can range from mild to severe.

What You Need to Know

- The most common causes of dehydration are diarrhea and vomiting. With diarrhea, stools will obviously be frequent and loose, but without diarrhea stools may be absent.
- Other causes are excessive sweating and urination. With a fever (see pages 146–49), the body loses extra fluid through the skin.
- Body fluids contain important salts and minerals that must be replaced along with water when a baby's dehydrated.
- Breastfed babies are less likely to develop dehydration, and breastfeeding should be continued during the illness.

Supplies

Thermometer, breast milk or other clear liquids (specifically oral rehydration solutions or electrolyte mixes)

Symptoms

- Very dry mouth and lips
- Sunken eyes and fontanel (soft spot on the head)
- Drowsiness
- Lack of energy
- Dry skin, wrinkled skin, or skin with a doughy texture
- Decreased urine output
- Decreased or absent tears when crying
- Fever (See pages 146–49.)
- Weight loss

Get Professional Help If:

- Your baby's symptoms are severe and he's either excessively sleepy or fussy.
- He has persistent vomiting or diarrhea (see pages 174–75) and can't keep down liquids.
- Home remedies don't improve his condition.
- He has diabetes and shows signs of dehydration.

What to Check

Is your baby urinating infrequently (no wet diapers in six hours or fewer than eight wet diapers in twenty-four hours)?

Treatment

Nurse your baby more often, or offer him more bottles of formula and clear liquids (preferably a commercially prepared electrolyte mix). If he is vomiting, give him one teaspoon (5 milliliters) of liquids at a time. Offer fluids frequently and increase the amount gradually as able. After he's vomited, let your baby rest before starting treatment. Your baby will need to consume extra fluids to compensate for the fluid lost in the diarrhea or vomiting. The total amount depends on his size.

Weight	Electrolyte Solution Amount
6–10 lb.	16 oz. per 24 hrs.
11–22 lb.	23 oz. per 24 hrs.
23–26 lb.	40 oz. per 24 hrs.

Diaper Rash

Description

Diaper rash appears on the skin that's covered by a diaper.

What You Need to Know

- Constant skin contact with urine and stool causes the rash. One simple cure: let your baby go diaper-free for a little while every day.
- Yeast (candida) is a common cause of persistent diaper rash and requires medication for treatment. If your baby's taking an antibiotic, he has an increased chance of getting a yeast infection.
- Plastic pants or tight disposable diapers can aggravate diaper rash.
- Most babies get some form of diaper rash before they're toilet trained. The peak age seems to be about eight to ten months.
- Diaper rash often occurs when a baby has diarrhea or when more frequent stools are passed.

Supplies

Water, a diaper rash ointment or cream, barrier jelly that's recommended by your baby's care provider

Symptoms

Redness or red patches, with or without tiny pimples, on skin that's covered by a diaper; open sores or blisters may develop in more severe cases.

Get Professional Help If:

- Your baby's diaper rash starts looking severe or pimples develop whiteheads or blisters.
- Home treatment fails to improve his rash in a few days.
- Fever is present.
- The rash is painful.

What to Check

Is your baby allergic to something that comes in contact with the affected skin? Possible allergens include plastic pants, disposable diapers, detergents, powders, lanolin, perfumes, alcohol, lotions, and fabric softeners.

Treatment

- Change your baby's diapers more frequently, and use plain water to carefully clean him after each change. If you use disposable wipes, they shouldn't contain fragrance or alcohol. Let the wet spots air-dry, or pat them dry before putting on a fresh diaper. Rubbing may be painful and may delay healing.
- Apply a thick layer of diaper rash ointment or cream, or barrier jelly, on the affected skin.
- If possible, let your baby go without a diaper for as long as possible.
- If a yeast infection is causing the rash, have your baby's care provider recommend a treatment.

Diarrhea

Description

Diarrhea causes frequent, loose, watery bowel movements that are yellowish, light brown, or green.

What You Need to Know

- Causes of diarrhea include bacteria, viruses, parasites, diet change, food, soy or milk intolerance or allergy, food poisoning, antibiotics, or viruses. Rotavirus is one of the most common causes of diarrhea during the first year. (An oral vaccination is available to help prevent this cause of diarrhea). It usually appears in the winter and often produces unusually foul-smelling stools. Infections outside the intestinal tract, such as ear, urine, and respiratory infections, can also present with diarrhea as a symptom.
- Breastfed infants normally will have up to twelve loose bowel movements each day in the first few months; this is not diarrhea.
- Diarrhea often accompanies colds, sore throats, or infections of the stomach and intestines.
- Diarrhea can cause dehydration, especially when accompanied by vomiting.

Supplies

Thermometer, breast milk or formula, and clear liquids (preferably a commercially prepared electrolyte mix)

Symptoms

- Liquid bowel movements
- More bowel movements than usual

Get Professional Help If:

- Your baby has loose bowel movements more than once every hour or two, for more than twelve hours.
- He has a fever of 102.5°F (39.2°C) or higher for more than one to two days. (See pages 146–49.)
- He has blood in his stools.
- He shows signs of dehydration. (See page 172.)
- He seems to be in pain.
- He has even mild diarrhea for more than two weeks.
- He refuses to eat or drink anything.

What to Check

- Are there signs of dehydration? (See page 172.)
- Is he urinating normally?
- How frequent are his bowel movements and what's their consistency?
- Has his diet changed recently?
- Does he have a fever? (See pages 146–49.)

Treatment

- If the diarrhea is mild (fewer than six to eight watery stools a day), you can usually keep your baby on his normal diet.
- For more severe diarrhea (or if vomiting accompanies the diarrhea), rest your baby's intestinal tract by withholding formula and solid foods for no more than twenty-four hours. You should try to continue breastfeeding.

- While his intestinal tract rests, frequently give your baby small amounts of breast milk or clear electrolyte solutions to satisfy thirst and prevent dehydration. (Don't use heavily sugared beverages like juice, and never use boiled skim milk.) Don't force him to drink the liquids, and don't withhold other foods longer than necessary—certainly not longer than twenty-four hours.

- After twenty-four hours of withholding solid foods (if your baby eats solids), begin feeding him rice, applesauce, pears, bananas, crackers, toast, flavored gelatin, or cereal. If you are formula feeding, you may want to temporarily use a soy formula. Diarrhea can shed the enzymes that normally help digest the milk sugar lactose.

- On the third day, resume his normal diet.

- Put zinc oxide or another type of topical barrier on the skin covered by a diaper, if it's sore.

- Never use over-the-counter antidiarrheal medications. They can actually worsen the diarrhea.

- You may want to discuss the use of prebiotics (natural food substances that promote a healthy intestinal lining) or probiotics ("friendly" bacteria) with your care provider.

Ear Infection
(Otitis Media)

Description

An ear infection appears as inflammation or accumulation of fluid in the middle ear, usually caused by bacterial or viral infection.

What You Need to Know

- Two out of three babies experience at least one ear infection by age two.

- Ear infections are most frequent between six months and three years of age. Boys have a higher frequency of ear infections than girls.

- A family history of ear infections makes a baby more susceptible.

- Colds often cause the Eustachian tubes (that connect the throat and nose and middle ear space) to swell and close, especially in babies. In babies, the Eustachian tube is shorter and positioned so that the nose and throat communicate easily with the middle ear space. Fluids build up in the middle ear, causing pain and sometimes temporary hearing loss.

- Ear infections occur more often in the winter and early spring.

- Day care attendance and exposure to secondhand smoke increase risk.

- A baby who drinks a bottle while lying flat on his back, or a breastfed baby nursed while lying on his side, may be at greater risk of developing an ear infection. Teach an older baby to use a sippy cup early on as a useful prevention.

- Keep your baby up to date on vaccines to help decrease the chance of ear infections.

Supplies

Thermometer, infant acetaminophen or ibuprofen (babies younger than six months should not take ibuprofen; see pages 147–48 for dosage information), prescribed ear drops, heating pad or hot-water bottle

Symptoms

- Chills and fever (See pages 146–49.)

- Congestion, runny nose

- Ear discharge (may be blood-tinged or yellow; results from a perforation of the eardrum that usually self-heals)

- Fussiness

- Inability to sleep

- Apparent hearing loss

- Rubbing/tugging at ear

- Crying during feeding

- Matter in eyes or discharge from eyes

Get Professional Help If:

- His temperature is higher than 101°F (38.3°C).

- Your baby tugs or rubs his ear(s) and he has other symptoms. (Some babies tug on their ears out of habit.)

- He has trouble balancing or develops an apparent hearing loss.

- He has yellow to red discharge draining from the ear. This may mean his eardrum has ruptured.

What to Check

Monitor your baby's fever.

Treatment

- Apply heating pad or hot water bottle to your baby's ear.
- Pain-relieving ear drops may be helpful in some circumstances. Check with your provider to see if these should be used.
- Avoid smoke exposure.
- Have your baby's care provider examine your baby, even if treatment relieves his pain. It's important to follow the findings. Many ear infections get better all by themselves. If it's suspected that bacteria has caused the infection, the care provider may prescribe antibiotics to clear the infection.

- Make sure you follow the medication instructions, even after your baby's symptoms subside.
- Give your baby infant acetaminophen or ibuprofen—check first with his care provider.
- To treat discharge, your care provider may prescribe antibiotic ear drops. Warm the bottle; lay your baby on his back with his head turned to his side, affected ear up; pull out, down, and back on the earlobe. Trickle ear drops into the ear so the liquid runs in.
- After an ear infection clears up, have the care provider check your baby for any complications that may have arisen. Persistent fluid and potential hearing problems need to be monitored.

Eczema
(Atopic Dermatitis)

Description

Eczema is an often inherited condition that's characterized by dry, red scaly skin and intense itching. These symptoms may be severe enough to interfere with eating and sleeping. The skin can be bumpy and moist at times. Eczema can present by one month of age and often improves by two to three years.

What You Need to Know

- Eczema's cause is unknown. Too-frequent bathing, an allergic reaction, or dry heat can trigger outbreaks. Heredity appears to play a strong role.
- Babies with eczema are also more likely to have food sensitivities, asthma, and allergies.
- Eczema often disappears with the use of proper lotions or creams.
- Infant eczema usually occurs on the face, in the bends of the elbows, and behind the knees. The diaper area is usually not affected.
- Touching an irritant or allergen can cause a similar-appearing type of rash at the site, called contact dermatitis. Contact dermatitis is treated much like eczema (with topical creams), but avoiding the irritant or allergen is important, too.

Supplies

Fragrance-free moisturizers, hydrocortisone ointment (prescription or over the counter), mild soap, cool-mist vaporizer or humidifier, baby nail clippers

Symptoms

- Pink or red rash
- Intense itching
- Irritability
- When scratched, a rash oozes a moist substance that dries and aggravates itching.

Get Professional Help If:

- Home treatment doesn't improve your baby's rash within a week.
- The rash appears infected.

What to Check

- Was a new food, clothing, or substance recently exposed to your baby's skin or environment?
- Is soap rinsed thoroughly from your baby's body after baths?
- Do other relatives have eczema?

Treatment

- Use mild soap and reduce the frequency and lengths of your baby's baths. Use fragrance-free moisturizers immediately after bathing your baby. Thick creams or ointments containing little to no water are preferred. Lotions are less effective. Keep the skin as hydrated as possible.

- Relieve your baby's itching with an over-the-counter hydrocortisone ointment or other topical medication.

- Cut your baby's fingernails (see page 42) to reduce irritation from scratching. Keep air moist with a cool-mist vaporizer or humidifier. Make sure you clean it every day.

- Eliminate aggravating factors such as heat, dryness in the environment, rapid temperature changes, and exposure to sensitizing chemicals and cleaning solutions.

- If a particular food is causing the eczema, eliminate it from your baby's diet, but don't change his diet extensively without his care provider's supervision.

- Avoid dressing your baby in wool clothing or in clothing made of other irritating fabrics.

- If the eczema is severe, your baby's care provider may suggest over-the-counter or prescription oral anti-itching medications.

Flat Heads
(Plagiocephaly, Positional Skull Deformity, Torticollis)

Description

The back of a baby's skull (the occiput) appears flattened or misshapen. This can involve the entire back of the head or one side more than the other.

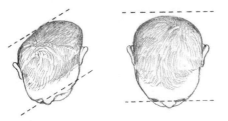

What You Need to Know

- Babies have soft, pliable skulls to allow for the important brain growth that continues to take place after birth. While in utero, the confines of the womb may make the skull asymmetrical. Tight neck muscles (torticollis) may also cause misshapen heads or heads that turn more one way than the other.

- The incidence of flat heads has increased significantly since experts began to recommend that babies sleep on their backs to help prevent Sudden Infant Death Syndrome (SIDS) in 1994. It's of utmost importance that babies remain on their backs while they sleep, but they should spend time on their stomachs ("tummy time") during the day to help develop their neck muscles and prevent flat heads.

- Brain growth and development are *not* affected by a misshapen head.

Supplies

Colorful toys and mobiles, CranioCap

Symptoms

The flattened area of your baby's head might not have as much hair growing over it as the rest of his scalp. Looking from above, his head may appear more diamond shaped than square. His neck muscles may be shorter or tighter on one side than the other.

Get Professional Help If:

- Flattening is not improving over the first few months or your baby cries and protests during attempts to turn his head in the other direction. Evaluation by four to six months of age is best.

- There is a ridge along a skull suture line or the skull is unusually long and thin, or flat and wide. This may indicate a rare early fusion of the skull bones called craniosynostosis, and require surgery.

What to Check

- Are you doing enough tummy time with your baby when he is awake?

- Are you placing various objects around your baby and positioning the crib so he is encouraged to look in different directions?

Treatment

- Reposition your baby often and be sure to practice "tummy time," but only when your baby is awake. The American Academy of Pediatrics (AAP) suggests starting with three to five minutes each day and gradually increasing the time he spends on his tummy, up to thirty minutes.

- Use colorful toys and mobiles to encourage your baby to move his head in more than one direction.

- Don't use wedges to position your baby's head. His head could get caught between the wedge and bed, causing suffocation.

- If your baby's neck muscles are tight, physical therapy can help relax them. See a trained specialist before you try anything at home.

- In more severe cases, a care provider may prescribe and fit a molding device or helmet (called a CranioCap) to be worn until your baby's head returns to an acceptable shape.

- The rare condition of craniosynostosis may require surgery.

Food Allergy

Description

An exaggerated response of the immune system to otherwise harmless proteins in foods indicates a food allergy. The reaction usually occurs within five minutes to one hour. The reaction reoccurs with each exposure to the food and can accompany eating, touching, or breathing the food.

What You Need to Know

- Food allergies are more common in children than adults, occurring in 2 to 8 percent of children under three years of age. Children often outgrow food allergies as their immune systems mature. The tendency to have food allergies is likely genetically inherited.
- Allergies are different from intolerances, sensitivities, or food poisoning.
- Cow's milk, eggs, and peanuts are the most common allergies in babies and children. Soy and wheat allergies are the next most common.
- It's not clear whether a breastfeeding mother can transfer allergy potential to her infant through the foods she ingests. If your baby has a reaction when you eat a certain food, avoid it.
- Delaying the introduction of solid foods until six months may help your baby avoid food allergies and allergic conditions like eczema and asthma. If your baby's digestive tract isn't mature enough, the large proteins found in solid foods can sometimes get through the lining of his intestinal wall. If this happens, his immune system kicks in

and produces antibodies, resulting in an allergic reaction.

- If your family has a history of allergies, you should not necessarily delay introducing these foods. Check with your care provider about your specific situation.

Supplies

Epinephrine auto-injector device, antihistamines

Symptoms

Symptoms may range from mild to severe and may involve the gastrointestinal, integumentary (skin), and respiratory systems.

- Gastrointestinal: vomiting, cramps, diarrhea
- Integumentary (skin): eczema, hives
- Respiratory: sneezing, wheezing
- Anaphylaxis (rare but life threatening): swelling of the tongue and throat, breathing trouble (may include wheezing), blue skin, decrease in blood pressure and weak pulse, loss of consciousness (See page 153 for more information.)

Get Professional Help If:

- You believe a reaction may be anaphylaxis. Call 911 immediately.
- You need help figuring out if a food allergy is present and how to avoid reactions in the future. Further allergy testing may be of help.

What to Check

How does your baby react after you introduce a new food?

Treatment

- Introduce solid foods one at a time. Wait at least two to four days after each new food to make sure it doesn't cause an allergic reaction. If your family has a history of allergies, wait a full week before offering the food again. Avoid stews, soups, or multigrain cereals; if any of these causes an allergic reaction in your baby, you won't know exactly which ingredient is to blame.

- If a food causes a reaction, avoid it. You can try serving the food again in very small amounts when your child is older, but only under the direction of a physician. You also can get blood or skin tests done to help evaluate allergies, though skin tests may be more helpful when your child is older than twelve months.

- If the food causes a severe reaction, your baby's care provider should prescribe an epinephrine auto-injector device and train you to use it in case of any food allergy resulting in an anaphylactic reaction. In an emergency, administer the medicine and call 911.

- If your baby needs an epinephrine auto-injector device, then he may need to wear a medical identification bracelet.

Gastroesophageal Reflux (GER) and Gastroesophageal Reflux Disease (GERD)
(Acid Reflux, Regurgitation, Spilling)

Description

Gastroesophageal reflux (GER) is when the stomach contents travel back into the esophagus (feeding tube) and possibly as far up as the mouth and nose. This occurs when the muscles at the junction of the esophagus and stomach (called the sphincter) do not close completely. Gastroesophageal reflux disease (GERD) occurs when GER causes severe symptoms or complications.

What You Need to Know

- Babies with GER often spit up (which leads many to call them "happy spitters"). This is a very common condition, because the sphincter muscles are often immature in young infants. Fifty percent of babies between one and three months of age throw up at least once a day. The spitting up often peaks when a GER baby is around four months old and stops most often when he's around ten months old—and almost always by his second birthday. GER babies may spit up less if their food is thickened (see treatment) or if they're kept upright for twenty to thirty minutes after feedings. Most GER babies outgrow their reflux without problems.

- Premature babies and babies who have a family history of GERD are at higher risk of developing the disease.

Supplies

The care provider may suggest thickening your baby's formula with baby cereal.

Symptoms

GER

- Spitting up

GERD

- Vomiting, possibly painful or forceful
- Cough
- Poor weight gain
- Abdominal or lower chest pain or tenderness
- Difficult or painful swallowing
- Heartburn (esophagitis)
- Respiratory problems including asthma and recurrent pneumonia
- Irritability
- Arching of the back
- Constipation or diarrhea

Get Professional Help If:

- Your baby vomits green or yellow material or blood.
- Your baby is gaining weight poorly.
- Irritability is significant.
- Vomiting is forceful and frequent, after most feedings. Your baby's care provider may need to evaluate for pyloric stenosis (a narrowing of the pylorus, the opening from the stomach into the small intestine).

What to Check

- Have your baby's care provider examine your baby if he has GER or GERD symptoms. Most times, a medical professional can diagnose GER or GERD by taking a careful history of the symptoms and thoroughly examining a baby to rule out other problems. In severe cases, he or she may do other diagnostic testing for further evaluation.

- Some babies who are allergic to cow's milk or soy may mimic GER or GERD symptoms. If your baby has blood in his stool, eczema, or if there is a strong family history of allergic disease, your baby will be at higher risk of having a cow's milk or soy allergy.

Treatment

- If your baby breastfeeds, continue nursing him. Most babies spit up breast milk less often than they do formula.

- If your baby consumes cow's milk or soy formula, his care provider may suggest giving him a cow's milk–free or hypoallergenic (hydrolyzed-protein) formula.

- Moms of breastfed infants may need to eliminate cow's milk and soy milk from their own diets.

- Avoid any exposure to smoke.

- If your baby is formula fed, adding infant cereal such as oat cereal to thicken his formula may help alleviate GER or GERD symptoms. One tablespoon of cereal to one ounce of milk is the recommended recipe. You can also buy formulas with premixed rice starch

for this purpose. Check with his care provider first.

- Keeping your baby upright for at least twenty to thirty minutes after eating, such as by holding him on your shoulder, often helps alleviate GER or GERD symptoms. Don't put your baby on his stomach to sleep—this position increases the risk of sudden infant death syndrome (SIDS) and puts pressure on your baby's belly.

- Placing your baby in a car seat or infant seat to keep him upright is not recommended. The "bent" position will put pressure on his belly and possibly aggravate GER or GERD symptoms.

- Don't overfeed your baby. Burp him often so gas won't put pressure on his belly. Keep his diaper and clothes loose at the waist.

- Your baby's care provider may prescribe a trial of acid-suppressant medications, which consist either of histamine H2-receptor antagonists or proton pump inhibitors.

- Surgery for GER and GERD is controversial and rarely needed except for severe cases.

Head Trauma/Injury
(Traumatic Brain Injury, Concussion)

Description

A minor head injury is an episode of blunt trauma to the scalp, skull, or brain in which the infant remains alert and awakens to light touch or voice. A traumatic brain injury is accompanied by signs that the brain is not functioning normally.

A concussion refers to a brief, temporary loss of consciousness following a hard knock or blow to the head. It is a subtype of a traumatic brain injury and a term that is not typically used with regard to infants.

What You Need to Know

- Minor head injuries are common and inevitable but rarely a cause for concern.
- Serious injuries can cause internal bleeding that puts pressure on the brain. Symptoms can appear even one to two days following the injury.
- If you suspect your infant's neck is seriously injured, do not move him unless absolutely necessary. Moving him could make the injury worse.
- Prevention by following safety guidelines (see Chapter 4) is preferable to dealing with the effects of an injury.
- Unfortunately, some injuries are inflicted by abuse of an infant—be on the alert for the possibility that your baby may have been the victim of an adult's or older child's anger or outburst.

Supplies

Ice, soap, and water

Symptoms

These symptoms will vary according to the severity and location of the injury.

- Some scalp bleeding, a "goose egg," crying up to ten minutes; these signs are common after a minor bump. There are lots of blood vessels on the scalp, so bumps appear more easily there.
- Odd behavior, giving a high-pitched cry, or loss of alertness; these are signs of a more serious injury.
- Vomiting
- Blood or bloody drainage coming from the nose or ears

Get Professional Help If:

- Your baby loses consciousness.
- After hitting his head, he cries and is inconsolable for more than ten minutes.
- He vomits more than twice.
- One of his pupils becomes larger than the other.
- He behaves abnormally, experiences a loss of coordination, shows any seizure activity, or is persistently irritable.
- He suffers a cut that's deep or bleeds a lot (it might need stitches).
- He has a larger than usual bump on his head.
- In an infant, it is best to be cautious; have him checked for anything more significant than a light bump.

What to Check

- How does your baby act? If the injury is serious, he'll most likely act abnormally.

- Watch him closely for twenty-four to forty-eight hours after the injury. If the blow was hard, your baby's care provider may advise that you wake your baby a few times during the night to check his behavior.

Treatment

- Watch your baby for abnormal behavior.

- Apply ice or a cold compress to the injured area for twenty minutes to relieve pain and reduce swelling.

- Wash cuts with soap and water. A deep or large cut may require stitches.

Hearing Loss

Description

A partial or total loss of hearing can be caused by a congenital defect, ear infections, illness, or injury. There are two main types of hearing loss: Conductive hearing loss results from problems in the outer or middle ear and is often medically or surgically treatable. Sensorineural loss (nerve deafness) comes from an inner ear problem or nerve problems between the inner ear and brain and is often permanent, though using a hearing aid may help.

What You Need to Know

- A sudden loss of hearing is usually temporary and probably means a foreign object, infection, or earwax is blocking the eardrum. (Letting some water get into your baby's ears during regular bathing can help prevent excessive earwax buildup.)
- Your baby may be at more risk of a sensorineural hearing loss if there's a history of deafness in your family.
- A baby needs to be able to hear in order to understand spoken language and, later, to produce clear speech. It's important to detect and diagnose hearing problems in order for a child to have normal language development.
- Mild hearing loss is common when a baby has a cold or allergies, because that's when fluid can accumulate in the middle ear space. This is usually temporary but should be monitored closely.

Supplies

None

Symptoms

Birth to Age Three Months

- Awakens to your touch but not to your voice
- Doesn't smile when spoken to
- Doesn't startle at loud noises
- Doesn't seem to recognize your voice or be calmed down by your voice when crying

Age Four to Six Months

- Doesn't try to turn toward a sound made at eye level
- Responds to comforting only when held
- Doesn't pay attention to music
- Shows little interest in babbling or imitating sounds
- Doesn't respond to speech sounds, footsteps, or noise-producing toys by stopping his activities to listen

Age Seven to Twelve Months

- Doesn't turn and look in the direction of sounds
- Doesn't respond when spoken to
- Ignores a ringing telephone or doorbell
- Seems startled to see a person nearby

Get Professional Help If:

- Your baby has any of the above symptoms.
- You have any reason to suspect that your baby has trouble hearing.

What to Check

- Was a newborn hearing test done before your baby left the hospital or birth center? If so, what were the results? (The majority of states mandate hearing screening be done before a newborn is discharged from the hospital.)
- Have you observed the startle reflex in your baby in response to loud noises? (See page 21.)
- Does your baby react when you squeeze a squeak toy near him?
- If you have any concerns about your baby's hearing, have his care provider schedule a formal hearing test with an audiologist.

Treatment

Have your baby's care provider:

- Treat all conditions that cause an ear infection or other suspected cause of hearing loss.
- Remove a foreign object from your baby's ear—do not remove the object yourself.
- Remove earwax buildup at your baby's next checkup; do not insert any object—even a cotton swab—into your baby's ear.
- Refer you to an ear, nose, and throat specialist for consideration of ear ventilation tube insertion, if persistent conductive hearing loss issues are of concern; you may also need to get a formal hearing evaluation from an audiologist to be able to accurately assess the hearing loss and decide if hearing aids are indicated. A surgery called a cochlear implant is another possible intervention for patients with sensorineural hearing loss.

Heat Rash/Sunburn

Description

Heat rash, also known as prickly heat or miliaria, appears as small red bumps in the folds of skin, especially on the neck and upper chest. Sunburn appears as red, painful skin and feels hot to the touch. Frequent sunburns are associated with an increased risk of skin cancer and premature aging.

What You Need to Know

- Heat rash is very common and causes only minor discomfort. It occurs most often in the summer, when it's humid, and can improve in a few hours or days.

- Heat rash is caused when pores that lead to sweat glands are blocked.

- Never leave a baby in a vehicle for even a few minutes, but especially not a closed one.

- The signs of sunburn show up six to twelve hours after exposure, and the pain is most severe in the first twenty-four hours.

- To prevent sunburn, dress your baby in long-sleeved clothing made of natural fibers and in a wide-brimmed hat. If your baby is six months or older, apply a PABA-free sunblock (at least SPF 30) that protects against both UVA and UVB rays. Midday sunlight is the strongest, so try not to expose your baby to the sun between 10 a.m. and 4 p.m.

- If your baby is less than six months old, it's best not to expose him to direct sunlight, and don't apply sunscreen at this age. If you cannot avoid being in the sun, use protective clothing and a sunscreen with an SPF of 15.

- A severe sunburn could lead to heatstroke, a serious condition. See page 192.

Supplies

Equipment needed for cool baths, thermometer

Symptoms

- Many tiny red bumps in folds of the skin, most often on cheeks, neck, shoulders, and diaper area (heat rash)

- Hot, red, painful skin (sunburn)

- Signs of dehydration, including decreased urine output, decreased or absent tears, dry lips and mouth, sunken soft spots, and lethargy (sunburn)

- Blisters, if severe

Get Professional Help If:

- Blisters appear on the bumps.

- Your baby develops a fever after being overheated.

- He has a sunburn that blisters.

What to Check

- Does your washing machine thoroughly rinse his clothing? Some detergents and bleaches aggravate heat rash.

- Is your baby overdressed? Excess clothing may contribute to heat rash.

- Are oily skin products blocking his pores?

- Does he have a fever? A sunburn with a fever may be an indication of heatstroke.

Treatment

- Move your baby to a cool place immediately.

- Keep your baby's skin as cool and dry as possible.

- Give frequent, cool baths or apply cool compresses to help open skin pores. Fanning him may help as well.

- Dress him in as little clothing as possible, and make sure the clothing is made of natural fibers. Put him in an air-conditioned environment or by a fan if possible.

- A severe sunburn should be treated the same as any burn: apply cold water or use a cold compress for fifteen minutes, then you may apply an aloe vera gel to help heal the skin.

- Give acetaminophen or ibuprofen as needed for pain (babies younger than six months should not take ibuprofen; see pages 147–48 for dosage information).

Heatstroke
(Heat Exhaustion)

Description

Heatstroke is a life-threatening condition that occurs when a person becomes excessively overheated. It's caused by external heat, not internal heat (fever). Heatstroke can occur when a baby is in a hot place, like a beach or a closed vehicle, for too long.

What You Need to Know

- Heatstroke is a medical emergency. Call 911 if you suspect your baby has heatstroke.

- Never leave a baby in a vehicle for even a few minutes, but especially not a closed one.

- To prevent sunburn (which can cause heatstroke), dress your baby in light long-sleeved clothing made of natural fibers and in a wide-brimmed hat. If your baby is more than six months old, apply a PABA-free sunblock (at least SPF 30). Midday sunlight is the strongest, so try not to expose your baby to the sun between 10 a.m. and 4 p.m.

Supplies

Equipment needed for cool baths, thermometer

Symptoms

- High fever (See pages 146–49.)
- Hot, red, dry skin
- Rapid pulse
- Restlessness

- Dizziness
- Vomiting
- Rapid, shallow breathing
- Unconsciousness
- Signs of dehydration, including decreased urine output, decreased or absent tears, dry lips and mouth, sunken soft spots, and lethargy

Get Professional Help If:

- Your baby develops a fever after being overheated.

- He has a sunburn that blisters.

What to Check

- Does he have a fever?
- Is he lethargic?
- Does he seem dehydrated?

Treatment

- Call 911 right away.

- Move your baby to a cool place immediately.

- Keep your baby's skin as cool and dry as possible.

- Give frequent cool baths or sponge baths. Fanning him may help as well.

- Dress him in as little clothing as possible, and make sure the clothing is made of natural fibers. Put him in an air-conditioned environment if possible.

Impetigo
(Pyoderma, Impetigo Contagiosa)

Description

Impetigo is a contagious bacterial infection of the skin, often around the nose, mouth, eyes, and ears. There is usually an underlying injury or irritation of the skin. This infection is more likely to occur in warm weather.

What You Need to Know

- Impetigo can spread rapidly from one part of the body to another or from person-to-person contact.
- Although not serious, impetigo must be treated persistently.

Supplies

Soap and water, compresses, antibiotic ointment or cream (prescription or over the counter), baby nail clippers

Symptoms

- Yellowish bumps or scabs on the skin, often in groups, with or without a honey-colored fluid or crust
- Possible blisters

Get Professional Help If:

- The infection spreads or doesn't respond to home treatment after five days.
- Your baby's urine turns red or brownish—a symptom of a rare kidney complication.

What to Check

- Because impetigo is contagious, check other family members for signs of infection.
- Make sure each family member uses his or her own towel and washcloth.

Treatment

- Gently clean the sores with soap and water, then put a compress on them for ten minutes.
- Gently rub away the crust and pus when the crust softens.
- Cover sores with over-the-counter antibiotic ointment or cream three times a day. Continue treatment three to four times a day until all sores lose their scabs. In severe cases, your baby's care provider may prescribe an oral or topical antibiotic.
- Loosely cover the sores with cloth to prevent spread (if the sores are not on baby's face).
- Clip your baby's nails (see page 42) to discourage scratching or playing with the bumps and scabs, which spreads the infection.
- A baby can return to day care after being on treatment for twenty-four hours.

Influenza
(Flu)

Description

A viral respiratory illness that may affect both the upper respiratory tract (nose and throat) and lower respiratory tract (bronchial tubes and lungs). It is more severe than the common cold and strikes almost every child from time to time. Distinct outbreaks occur and vary every year.

What You Need to Know

- Symptoms can include nausea, vomiting, and abdominal pain. Influenza should not be confused with gastroenteritis (commonly called stomach flu), with its main symptoms of vomiting and diarrhea.

- Influenza is highly contagious; it's spread by droplets that are coughed and sneezed into the air and by touching a contaminated surface or object. It is most frequent in the winter and early spring.

- There are subtypes of influenza, with A and B types responsible for most infections. The terms avian flu and swine flu or H1N1 refer to types of influenza that fall within the type A and B categories.

- New vaccines are made yearly to protect against the predicted strains. Babies are eligible for the vaccine beginning at six months.

- Young infants are at increased risk for complications and hospitalization for influenza. Household contacts should be vaccinated as well.

Supplies

If your baby is in pain or discomfort and/or has a high fever, give acetaminophen or ibuprofen to comfort him. (Babies younger than six months should not take ibuprofen.) See pages 147–48 for dosage information.

Symptoms

- High fever of 103°F to 105°F (39.4°C to 40.6°C); see pages 146–49.
- Chills and sweating
- Decreased energy
- Dry cough
- Runny or stuffy nose
- May be accompanied by ear infections, croup, bronchiolitis, and pneumonia and secondary vomiting and diarrhea
- Symptoms may last for more than a week.
- Some infants show very few symptoms.

Get Professional Help If:

- You suspect your baby has influenza. Contact your care provider early in the illness, as a prescribed antiviral medication may shorten the course of the illness and help prevent the spread of infection to others.

- Your baby has underlying health problems, such as heart or lung disease, a weakened immune system or a malignancy. There is increased risk of severe complications from influenza.

- There are signs of secondary infection such as ear pain, persistent cough or a cough that turns phlegmy, or sharp pain with breathing. Your care provider may need to prescribe antibiotics.

What to Check

Watch for difficulty breathing or a bluish color to your baby's skin. If either occurs, call 911.

Treatment

- Encourage good fluid intake and monitor for signs of dehydration, including decreased urine output, decreased or absent tears, dry lips and mouth, sunken soft spots, and lethargy.

- Once your baby is six months old, he can receive the influenza vaccine. See page 143 for more information.

- Your baby can return to day care once he is free of fever for twenty-four hours.

Meningitis

Description

A rare, serious disease in which a bacteria or virus inflames and infects the tissues surrounding the brain and spinal cord. There is about a 5 percent mortality rate from meningitis.

What You Need to Know

- A medical professional should diagnose and treat meningitis as soon as possible.
- Good hygiene, like frequent hand washing, can help prevent the spread of meningitis.
- Vaccinations can help prevent the most serious cases of meningitis. Make sure your baby is up to date on his immunizations.
- Babies less than two months of age are at higher risk of serious consequences from meningitis because of their less mature immune systems.

Supplies

Thermometer

Symptoms

- Moderate to high-grade fever (See pages 146–49.)
- Vomiting
- Decreased appetite
- Extreme listlessness or irritability, or extreme sleepiness
- Stiff neck (babies sometimes don't have this symptom)
- Sometimes, purple spots on body
- Bulging soft spot on head
- Seizures

Get Professional Help If:

- Your baby is less than two months old and has a fever.
- Your baby has meningitis symptoms. No single symptom suggests the disease; look for a combination of the above symptoms.
- You're unsure whether your baby has meningitis symptoms.

What to Check

Do you know whether your baby has been exposed to meningitis? Meningitis is often spread like a cold virus, but it can be spread through contact with stool, such as during diaper changes.

Treatment

Meningitis is a serious disease that always requires medical care. See your baby's care provider immediately if you suspect your baby has meningitis.

- A spinal tap (also called a lumbar puncture or LP) is necessary to confirm a diagnosis. This test involves using a special needle inserted into the lower back to obtain a sample of spinal fluid. Blood testing will also be done.
- Hospital admission and intravenous (IV) antibiotics, along with early diagnosis, usually result in full recovery.
- Babies that have had meningitis need to be followed up closely after infection for possible complications.

Pinkeye
(Conjunctivitis)

Description

Pinkeye is an irritation or infection (viral or bacterial) of the white part of the eye and the inside of the eyelid.

What You Need to Know

- An eye infected with pinkeye will have discharge as well as be bloodshot and pinkish.
- Pinkeye can be very contagious.
- Pinkeye is not the only cause of red eyes and discharge. Other possibilities include allergies, colds, chlorinated swimming pool water, dust, and injury to the eye.
- Babies with blocked tear ducts may be more susceptible to eye infections. If your baby has discharge in his eyes and sticky eyelashes, see his care provider to learn whether he needs prescribed antibiotics.
- Ear infections often accompany pinkeye.
- Pinkeye occurring in the newborn period can be caused by infections the mother may have caught during sexual activity. Drops administered right after birth will help prevent this form of infection.

Supplies

Prescribed antibiotics, cotton balls

Symptoms

- Red eyes, possibly painful and itchy
- Discharge from the eyes, often more abundant after sleep

- Swelling of eyelids
- Crying, irritability

Get Professional Help If:

- Your baby has irritated or swollen eyes, and you're not sure of the cause.
- Your baby has recurrent eye irritations or discharge.
- There is suspicion of an ear infection.

What to Check

- Has your baby had contact with someone with pinkeye?
- Has he had increased tearing since birth in one or both eyes?

Treatment

- Some forms of pinkeye require prescription antibiotic eye ointment or drops.
- To wipe away discharge from your baby's eyes, use a cotton ball that's dampened with clean water. Dispose of the cotton ball after each wipe over the eye.
- Wash your baby's hands frequently, and wash your hands after touching someone with pinkeye. Sanitize objects that are frequently touched such as doorknobs, cell phones, and toys.
- To protect other family members, keep your baby's washcloth and towel separate from other clothing.
- Discourage your baby from rubbing his eyes.

Pneumonia

Description

Pneumonia is an infection of the lungs, usually viral but sometimes bacterial.

What You Need to Know

- Pneumonia has several different causes, and its severity can vary greatly.
- Some forms of pneumonia are contagious; others aren't.
- Pneumonia occurs most commonly when a viral cold spreads into the lungs.
- It is most frequent in the fall, winter, and early spring.
- Going out in the cold does *not* cause pneumonia.
- Pneumonia is more likely to occur if the immune system is weakened or there is an underlying lung abnormality.
- Some types of pneumonia are prevented by vaccinations. Make sure your baby's immunizations are up to date.

Supplies

Thermometer, prescribed antibiotics (for some pneumonia), infant acetaminophen or ibuprofen (babies younger than six months should not take ibuprofen; see pages 147–48 for dosage information)

Symptoms

- Cough
- Fever (see pages 146–49) with sweating or chills
- Apparent stomach or chest pain
- Fast or labored breathing, possibly accompanied by flaring nostrils or wheezing
- "Sucked in" appearance of the breathing muscles between and below the ribs and above the collarbone
- Decreased appetite
- Possible vomiting
- A bluish tint to lips or nails may indicate decreased oxygen flow in the blood.

Get Professional Help If:

You suspect your baby has pneumonia. His care provider will diagnose the cause of the infection and may prescribe treatment, possibly with antibiotics. The care provider may x-ray your baby's chest to confirm the diagnosis. If your baby is very ill, he may need to be hospitalized. If he is not getting better or is showing signs of infection anywhere else in the body, he should be followed closely.

What to Check

- Does your baby have trouble breathing?
- Does he have a fever?

Treatment

- If your baby's care provider diagnoses pneumonia, he or she may decide to treat your baby with antibiotics.
- Rest is important; make sure your baby gets lots.
- Don't use a cough suppressant. Coughing helps move and clear the secretions associated with pneumonia.
- If your baby has a fever, give him infant acetaminophen or ibuprofen. (See pages 147–48 for dosage information.) Contact his care provider if the fever is persistent.

Poisoning, from Food

Description

Food poisoning typically occurs when your baby has eaten (or drunk) something that was contaminated with one of several dangerous bacteria. (These bacteria are sometimes transmitted by other people and animals.)

What You Need to Know

- Symptoms often do not appear until a couple of hours to two days later.
- Oftentimes the symptoms are mistaken for gastroenteritis (commonly called stomach flu).
- Symptoms typically last one or two days but sometimes last as long as a week or two.

Supplies

Breastmilk or formula, commercially prepared electrolyte solution (if instructed to give), thermometer

Symptoms

- Abdominal pain, cramps, and diarrhea
- Nausea and vomiting
- Excessive fussiness
- Tiny pink spots on skin
- Sometimes fever
- Rarely, blood in his stools

Get Professional Help If:

- Your baby has blood in his stool.
- Your baby has a high fever.
- Your baby has been vomiting for three or more days.
- Your baby becomes dehydrated.
- Your baby has a hard, swollen belly.

What to Check

- Excessive vomiting, which can lead to dehydration
- Listlessness from severe poisoning

Treatment

- If your baby has trouble breathing, swallowing, has sunken eyes, cold splotchy hands and feet, or is unresponsive, call 911.
- Don't make your baby vomit unless instructed to do so.
- Make sure you baby drinks breastmilk or formula; you may need to feed in frequent, small amounts.
- Your care provider may suggest offering an oral electrolyte solution for rehydration (not juice or soda).

Poisoning, from Toxic Substances

Description

Swallowing, breathing in, or making skin contact with certain medicines, cleaning products, petroleum-based products, or other toxic substances can cause poisoning. Half of all poisonings occur in children less than six years of age.

What You Need to Know

- Medicines, cleaners, houseplants, and other common items are the main causes of poisoning. (See page 115.)
- Safe storage can prevent poisoning, but be ready for emergencies by posting the phone number of the national poison control center (800-222-1222) near every telephone. Prevention information is available at http://www.poisonhelp .hrsa.gov.
- Some infants will have no symptoms early on but still may be in severe danger; get professional help if you suspect your baby has swallowed or put any toxic substance in his mouth.

Supplies

Water or milk (if instructed to give)

Symptoms

- Abdominal pain, cramps, and diarrhea
- Blackouts and unconsciousness
- Convulsions or seizures
- Choking or difficulty breathing
- Confusion and drowsiness
- Nausea, vomiting, and coughing up blood
- Behavior change
- Rash or burns, especially on the lips or mouth
- Excessive drooling or a strange odor on the breath
- Throat pain
- Stains on clothing without an apparent explanation

Get Professional Help If:

You suspect your baby has swallowed or put any toxic substance in his mouth.

What to Check

- Have any medicines, cleaners, or other harmful substances been opened, or are any missing?
- If you find your baby near an empty or open container of a dangerous substance, suspect poisoning.
- Does your home have lead-based paint in it? Lead-based paint chips can poison a baby who swallows them. (See page 115.)

Treatment

- Get the poisonous substance away from your baby. If some of the substance is in his mouth, try to help him spit it out or try to remove it with your fingers. Keep this material if you are not sure of the source.

- Call the national poison control center (800-222-1222) immediately. Be ready to give your name and phone number, your baby's name, age and weight, the name of the poisonous substance, and the time and amount you think was swallowed. Also share any medical conditions or medications your baby has.

- Don't make your baby vomit unless instructed to do so.

- If your baby has a poisonous substance on his skin, remove clothing and rinse the skin with room-temperature water.

- If your baby has a poisonous substance in his eye, hold his eyelid open and pour a steady stream of room-temperature water into the inner corner of the eye. Wrap your baby in a towel to help secure him if no one else is available to help hold him securely.

- If you or your baby is exposed to toxic fumes, get into fresh air immediately and then call for help.

- Take the container of the substance and a sample of any vomit to the emergency room with your baby. Make sure you keep both safely away from him.

Roseola
(Roseola Infantum, Exanthema Subitum)

Description

Roseola is marked by a fever and subsequent pinkish-red, blotchy rash; it is usually caused by a virus called human herpesvirus 6 (HHV-6).

What You Need to Know

- Roseola is common in babies seven to thirteen months old.
- There's no prevention or cure, but it is benign and self-limited and disappears on its own.
- The roseola rash usually appears after three to seven days of moderate to high-grade fever (see pages 146–49).
- Your baby is usually well when the rash disappears, within two days after it first appears. By that point, he is likely not contagious.

Supplies

Thermometer, infant acetaminophen or ibuprofen (babies younger than six months should not take ibuprofen; see pages 147–48 for dosage information), equipment for cool baths

Symptoms

- A high-grade fever of 103°F to 105°F (39.4°C to 40.6°C). (See pages 146–49.) Rarely, convulsions may accompany high-grade fever.
- Decreased appetite
- Mild crankiness or increased sleepiness
- A slight cough, runny nose, or diarrhea may be present.

- Slightly raised, distinct red spots
- Rash generally appearing on trunk, upper arms, and neck
- The rash appears after the fever disappears.
- Your baby may not appear sick or ill at all.
- The incubation period is seven to fourteen days. Once the fever is gone for twenty-four hours, your baby should no longer be contagious.

Get Professional Help If:

- The rash seems especially severe.
- Coughing, vomiting, or diarrhea accompany roseola symptoms.
- Low-grade fever lasts longer than four days without other symptoms.

What to Check

Any high-grade fever requires close observation. Roseola can be diagnosed only when the rash appears. If the rash doesn't appear, something else caused the fever and complications could have already occurred.

Treatment

- Treat your baby's fever. (See pages 146–49.) Dress your baby in light clothing.
- Watch your baby closely for other symptoms.
- Permit moderate activity if your baby feels like moving about.
- Hand washing may help prevent spread of infection.

Seizures
(Convulsions, Fits, Epilepsy)

Description

Seizures or convulsions are sudden events caused by abnormal electrical impulses and chemical changes in the brain that result in a temporary change in movement or behavior. A series of involuntary muscle spasms may make the body stiffen. In babies, convulsions may be more subtle. Epilepsy is a condition of repeated seizures that are not provoked by illness or injury.

What You Need to Know

- A convulsion is usually not life threatening. Most appear with fever (especially in children up to age three but rarely after age six). Fever-related convulsions (febrile seizures) usually end within a few minutes and don't cause permanent damage.

- Fever-related seizures usually occur when there is a family history of this condition, and they can recur in the early years. They usually occur early on in a febrile illness, sometimes even before you realize your baby is ill. Even diligent antifever measures might not prevent them. They are harmless and common. Most of the fevers are caused by viral infections. Roseola and influenza are more likely to be associated with seizures than other viruses.

- Most seizures of any kind will stop on their own.

- Other less common causes of convulsions include poisoning, severe infection, injury, and epilepsy. If epilepsy is diagnosed, antiseizure (anticonvulsant) medication may be prescribed.

Supplies

To treat a fever: Thermometer, cool water and washcloth, infant acetaminophen suppository

Symptoms

- Bluish face and lips
- Uncontrolled jerking or twitching body movements; rigidity or stiffness
- Vomiting or drooling
- Rolling eyes
- Fever might be present.
- Unresponsiveness
- Your baby just doesn't look "right."

Get Professional Help If:

- This is your baby's first convulsion. It's okay to call 911 for any convulsion, but it usually will have stopped by the time help arrives.

- A convulsion lasts more than a few minutes or is especially severe. Call 911 for any convulsion lasting more than fifteen minutes.

What to Check

- How does your baby act before and after convulsions?
- How long did the convulsion last?
- Did the convulsion affect one or both sides of his body?
- Is there a fever (see pages 146–49), or are there symptoms of infection or poisoning (see pages 199-201)? Has there been any recent head injury?

Treatment

- Place your baby on the floor or on a bed. Remove objects that may injure him. Try to remain calm, knowing the seizure will likely stop on its own.
- Turn him on his side with his hips higher than his head to prevent him from choking on vomit or saliva.
- Loosen any tight clothing.
- Don't place anything in his mouth, like tongue depressors, fingers, liquids, or medication while he's convulsing. He will not swallow his tongue.
- Once the convulsion is over, treat a fever as you normally would, or give your baby an infant acetaminophen suppository.
- Get medical help. If fever is present, your baby will need to be examined to determine the cause, including the possibility of meningitis.

Sudden Infant Death Syndrome
(SIDS, Cot or Crib Death)

Description

The sudden and unexplained death of an apparently normal, healthy baby during sleep for unknown reasons. There are about 2,500 deaths from SIDS each year in the United States.

What You Need to Know

- SIDS most often occurs when babies are between two and four months old, but almost always between one month and one year of age.

- SIDS is more common in boys than girls. Premature infants, low-birth-weight infants, multiples, those with a family history of SIDS, and those whose mothers smoke are also at risk. SIDS is less common in breastfed infants.

- To decrease the frequency of SIDS, the American Academy of Pediatrics (AAP) recommends that babies sleep on their backs. Research indicates that fewer SIDS deaths (about 50 percent) occur when babies sleep exclusively on their backs.

- A disproportionate number of SIDS deaths, about one in five cases, happen in day cares. Always make sure your child care providers—including baby-sitters—put your baby on his back to sleep. Babies who are "unaccustomed" to sleeping on their tummies because they are put to sleep on their backs by their parents and then suddenly put to sleep on their tummies by others have an eighteenfold chance of SIDS.

- It isn't conclusive if swaddling a baby has an effect on the incidence of SIDS. Some believe it helps prevent SIDS by keeping a baby on his back, but others think it may actually increase the risk, as it can be more difficult to wake up a swaddled baby if he isn't used to the practice. If your baby is swaddled early and safely and is not trying to turn, swaddling is likely safe.

- Once your baby learns to roll repeatedly from his back to his belly, it's okay to let him sleep on his stomach. But he should still be placed on his back to begin sleep.

- Pacifiers that are used to help your baby fall asleep may reduce the incidence of SIDS. Once your baby has fallen asleep, however, you should not reintroduce the pacifier. Make sure you've established breastfeeding before you introduce a pacifier.

- Vaccines do not cause SIDS and indeed may have a protective effect. Make sure your baby's immunizations are up to date.

- Vomiting does not cause SIDS. Always put your baby on his back to sleep.

- Baby monitors can alert you if your baby is crying but not if he's in danger of SIDS; even if you have a monitor, make sure you follow all other recommendations.

- Don't use wedges, positioners, or specialized sleep surfaces as they have not been found to decrease SIDS and may increase the risk of suffocation.

- Altitudes higher than eight thousand feet may pose a higher risk for SIDS.

Supplies

A sleeping area that has a firm surface, meets safety guidelines, and is free of thick blankets, stuffed animals, pillows, and so on. Cribs need to be safety approved and sheets need to be well fitting. Try not to use blankets and certainly never put them over your baby's head. If you do use blankets, they must be light and tucked in on all sides on the bottom half of the crib mattress. Do not use bumper pads, waterbeds, sheepskin bedding, or polystyrene-filled cushions for sleep. Having your baby sleep in the same room as you in a bassinet or crib could reduce his risk of SIDS, but having your baby sleep in the same bed as you could increase the risk. See the section on sleeping in Chapter 2 about the safest place for your baby to sleep.

Symptoms

None

Get Professional Help If:

- Your baby has sleep apnea—periods of twenty seconds or more when breathing stops.
- Your baby turns blue while sleeping.

What to Check

- Is your baby's mattress too soft? Soft surfaces and bedding may increase risk.
- Is your baby in a smoke-free environment? Are alcohol and drug use being avoided by caretakers in order to provide safe care?
- Is your baby's sleeping area too warm? Make sure the temperature is one in which you'd feel comfortable sleeping with light clothes on. If your baby sweats, has flushed cheeks, heat rash, or rapid breathing, the room is likely too warm.
- Make sure that if your baby inadvertently falls asleep in a car seat, stroller, swing, infant carrier, or sling that you move him to a firm, flat surface to continue sleeping.

Treatment

None. Parents of SIDS victims should contact their health care provider to find local support.

Teething

Description

The emergence and eruption of teeth (beginning around three to seven months of age) can cause tenderness of the gums, often accompanied by drooling.

What You Need to Know

- Not all babies teethe at the same time. (See pages 144–45.) Your baby's teething schedule will be different from any other baby's.
- Never let your baby go to sleep with a bottle of milk or any liquid containing sugar. These increase the risk of tooth decay when coating the teeth during sleep.

Supplies

Thermometer, infant acetaminophen or ibuprofen (babies younger than six months should not take ibuprofen; see pages 147–48 for dosage information), teething objects (rings, pacifiers, biscuits, and toys)

Symptoms

- Fussiness or crankiness
- Drooling
- Chewing fingers or other objects
- Crying
- Low-grade fever, usually less than 100°F (37.8°C) (See pages 146–49.)
- Tender, swollen gums
- Irritability
- Loose stools may accompany teething.

Get Professional Help If:

Signs of illness, like vomiting, accompany teething symptoms. Signs of appearing significantly ill should not be misinterpreted as teething. Teething shouldn't cause a high-grade fever; if your baby has one, consider other causes and, if necessary, contact your baby's care provider for a diagnosis and treatment.

What to Check

Consider other causes of your baby's symptoms—hunger, thirst, boredom, ear infection, a need for attention.

Treatment

- You can't do much to ease your baby's teething discomfort, but rubbing his gums with a clean finger may help. Hugs and kisses work as well as anything else.
- If your baby is weaning well and suddenly suffers from teething, he'll probably want to nurse or drink from the bottle instead of a cup. Don't deny him this comfort while he's miserable. When he starts to feel better, you can resume weaning.
- To relieve gum soreness, give your baby infant acetaminophen or ibuprofen. (See pages 147–48 for dosage information.)
- Offer your baby teething rings, pacifiers, biscuits, or toys to gnaw on. (See Chapter 5 for more information on teething toys.) Do not dip the teething toys in sugary substances (it can cause tooth decay). Teething items can be chilled but should not be frozen and should be one piece only to avoid choking. It is not recommended to use necklaces of any kind for teething.

- Avoid giving your baby topical over-the-counter medications that claim to relieve teething pain; their effectiveness hasn't been proven. Medications that you rub on your baby's gums may numb the back of the throat if overused, which could interfere with your baby's normal gag reflex.

- Once they've erupted, clean your baby's teeth with a soft, infant toothbrush or wipe them with gauze.

Thrush

Description

Thrush is a superficial infection of the mouth and tongue caused by the fungus candida (yeast).

What You Need to Know

- Thrush's only signs are white patches on the inside of the mouth, on the tongue and throat. They may disappear if ignored, but most parents want to treat them. The patches are usually irregularly shaped.
- Some babies may be fussy or have trouble feeding, though this is unusual.
- Thrush occurs more commonly in infants less than six months old, when the immune system is not fully developed.
- Thrush can be more frequent with regular pacifier use.
- A diaper rash caused by yeast may accompany the oral thrush.
- Thrush is not spread from baby to baby, so isolation is unnecessary.

Supplies

Prescribed medication, usually a topical antifungal medication

Symptoms

- White, creamy patches on the insides of the cheeks, behind the lips, or on the tongue
- Although they may look like dried or curdled milk, the patches don't wipe off as milk would.

Get Professional Help If:

Your baby has thrush or you suspect he does—although thrush isn't an urgent condition.

What to Check

Are there blisters inside your baby's mouth? If so, he may have some other condition.

Treatment

- If your baby's care provider has prescribed medication, apply it to the patches as directed.
- If you're breastfeeding your baby, you may need to apply medicated ointment to your nipples to prevent passing the infection back to your baby. (See page 81.) If you're bottle feeding your baby, sterilize all bottle nipples to prevent reinfection.
- If your baby uses a pacifier or teething rings or toys, thoroughly clean them with hot water daily while treating thrush.

Urinary Tract Infection (UTI)

Description

An infection of the urinary system (the kidneys, bladder, and their connecting structures—the ureters and urethra) can lead to various problems or can be a symptom of other illnesses. There are two main subtypes of urinary tract infections: pyelonephritis, when the infection involves the kidneys; and cystitis, when it involves the bladder. Infants are at high risk of getting pyelonephritis, which if not treated can lead to kidney damage.

What You Need to Know

- Urinary tract infections can be challenging to detect and treat, especially in babies. Fever may be the only symptom.
- UTIs may develop when part of the urinary tract does not form correctly during pregnancy.
- As newborns, boys and girls can get UTIs. Uncircumcised boys are at higher risk of getting a urinary tract infection. When older, girls are more at risk. Wiping only from the front to the back at diaper change may help decrease the chance of getting an infection.
- In infants less than one month, a UTI is often a part of a wider systemic infection, which is a much more serious situation.
- If there's no other cause of persistent high-grade fevers, a health care provider will often look for a UTI.

- Babies who have had a UTI are at a slightly higher risk of getting another infection.
- In older infants, symptoms of constipation may be similar to those of a bladder infection.

Supplies

Thermometer, infant acetaminophen or ibuprofen (babies younger than six months should not take ibuprofen; see pages 147–48 for dosage information), fluids

Symptoms

- Frequent, painful, or bloody urination
- Foul-smelling urine
- Apparent abdominal or back pain
- Fever (See pages 146–49.)
- Nausea
- Jaundice
- Possible vomiting
- Poor feeding and growing

Get Professional Help If:

- You detect any sign of urinary tract infection or blockage such as pain accompanying urination or back pain.
- Your baby has a fever higher than 100.4°F (38°C) or appears very ill.

What to Check

If there's a family history of bladder or kidney problems, let your baby's care provider know.

Treatment

- Until you see your baby's care provider, give your baby infant acetaminophen or ibuprofen for pain (see pages 147–48 for dosage information) and give him lots of fluids to keep flushing out his system.

- Your baby's care provider will test a urine sample to confirm whether your baby has an infection. This may involve inserting a catheter (a small tube) through the urethra into the bladder or inserting a needle through the skin and into the bladder to obtain a specimen for culture. If he has a bacterial UTI, further tests will likely be done to determine any underlying causes. The care provider will prescribe an antibiotic if he or she detects a bacterial infection. For young infants, this antibiotic is often given intravenously in a hospital.

Vomiting

Description

Vomiting, or the forceful expelling of stomach contents through the nose and mouth, is a common symptom with many causes.

What You Need to Know

- By far, the most common cause of vomiting is a contagious viral infection in the stomach.

- Infections outside the gastrointestinal tract such as respiratory infections (ear infections, pneumonia), urinary tract infections, poisoning, or meningitis may also cause vomiting. (See page 151 for cross references.)

- Noninfectious conditions including obstructions, increased pressure in the brain, and metabolic problems are much less common but can also cause vomiting. These require further medical evaluation.

- Frequent hand washing is the most effective way to prevent the spread of viral infections.

- Babies often spit up. Spitting up is not vomiting. With spitting up, the stomach contents come up easily and often accompany a burp.

- Dehydration is the main concern with vomiting.

- A baby's vomiting in the first few months may have some specific underlying causes:
  - If it occurs less than fifteen to thirty minutes after every feeding, he may have pyloric stenosis, an obstructive condition in which food can't pass out of the stomach into the small intestine. This condition is usually diagnosed between two and six weeks of age and requires surgery.
  - Muscles at the entrance to the stomach may be especially relaxed, resulting in a condition called gastroesophageal reflux (or GER) that allows upward movement of the stomach contents into the mouth. If symptoms accompany reflux (gastroesophageal reflux disease [GERD]), there are various treatments for this condition. (See pages 184–85.)

Supplies

Thermometer; clear liquids, preferably commercially prepared oral electrolyte solutions

Get Professional Help If:

- Any vomiting doesn't stop within twenty-four hours (twelve hours in a newborn) or is combined with drowsiness, irritability, apparent severe abdominal pain, high fever (see pages 146–49), or labored breathing.

- Vomit is bloody, or yellow or green (called bile), more than once or twice.

- Your baby forcefully vomits shortly after being fed.

- Your baby completely refuses to eat or drink anything after a few hours.

- The vomiting is accompanied by any appearance of blood in the stool.

What to Check

Look for signs of dehydration: listlessness, dry mouth, sunken eyes or soft spot, crying without tears, infrequent urination.

Treatment

- Closely watch your baby when he's vomiting, especially if he's younger than five months. Call his care provider if vomiting persists.

- A short time after he vomits, offer your baby one teaspoon to one tablespoon (4.9 to 14.8 milliliters) of breast milk or oral electrolyte solution every few minutes. Your provider can recommend which are the best electrolyte solutions. Do not use juices or other high-sugar-containing liquids. Do not use chicken broth—it has a high fat content and may be hard to digest.

- Gradually give him more clear liquids. Offer them frequently. Do not force him to eat or drink.

- Once the clear liquids are being retained, you may begin to offer solid foods slowly. Offer a variety of foods and follow your infant's cues as to what he is interested in. Continue to monitor hydration closely.

Whooping Cough
(Pertussis)

Description

Whooping cough is a highly contagious respiratory-tract bacterial infection, with a severe cough, that causes irritation and narrowing of the airway passages (bronchioles and bronchi). It can be very serious for babies who develop pneumonia or have trouble breathing. Whooping cough can be greatly diminished with the vaccine DTaP.

What You Need to Know

- Babies under six months of age and babies who have not received all of their vaccines (up through six months) are more likely to catch whooping cough and have complications from whooping cough.
- Make sure you, your family, and your baby's day care provider are all up to date on your vaccines. If you were not up to date, your health care provider most likely gave you a Tdap shot in your third trimester. This helped protect your newborn until he was able to get his shots.
- The coughing fits may last three months.

Supplies

Fluids: breastmilk, formula and water, chicken broth and vegetable broth for children over six months; vitamins C and D, plus probiotics (may help speed recovery)

Symptoms

- Typically starts off with common cold symptoms (cough, runny nose or congestion, sneezing, and maybe a fever)
- After a week or two, the cough changes to severe hacking coughing fits followed by a high-pitched intake of breath that sounds like "whoop." Many babies are not able to catch their breath, so they stop breathing.
- If coughing is forceful enough, it may trigger vomiting.

Get Professional Help If:

- Your baby has cold symptoms but after a week the cough gets worse, shows exhaustion after cough episodes, has problems eating, or appears very "sick."
- Your baby seems to be struggling to breathe, turns red or blue.
- The coughing is causing your baby to vomit.

What to Check

- Watch for breathing difficulty, especially during a coughing fit.
- Watch for dehydration or weight loss.
- Track if there has been any exposure to anyone with an especially bad or persistent cough.
- Take his temperature every four to six hours. (See page 149.)
- Follow closely if the cough is getting better, worse, or staying the same.

Treatment

- A test will be done to confirm diagnosis.
- Antibiotics will likely be given, especially if the diagnosis is made early on in the illness; they may lessen the duration and contagiousness.
- Most babies under six months are treated in the hospital.
- Your baby needs to stay away from people (outside of the immediate family) until his care provider has approved his integration, typically after one to three weeks (depending on whether antibiotics are given).
- There is very little you can do to relieve the cough, and it is not recommended to use medications, since they have very little effect on whooping cough.
- Get plenty of rest.
- Drink plenty of fluids.
- A cool-mist humidifier may soothe irritation. Make sure you clean it daily.
- If your baby is over six months old, give him small snacks rather than full meals.
- Complications of whooping cough can include seizures and pneumonia.
- Vitamins C and D, plus probiotics (may help speed recovery)

Appendix

Guide to Resources

Books

Agnew, Connie, Alan Klein, and Jill Alison Ganon. *Twins! Pregnancy, Birth, and the First Year of Life.* 2006.

American Academy of Pediatrics, The. *Caring for Your Baby and Young Child: Birth to Age 5.* 2014.

Brott, Armin A. *The New Father: A Dad's Guide to the First Year.* 2015.

Huggins, Kathleen. *The Nursing Mother's Companion: Revised Edition.* 2015.

Klaus, Marshall and Phyllis Klaus. *Your Amazing Newborn.* 2000.

La Leche League International. *The Womanly Art of Breastfeeding.* 2010.

Leach, Penelope. *Your Baby and Child: From Birth to Age Five.* 2010.

Lothian, Judith and Charlotte DeVries. *The Official Lamaze Guide: Giving Birth with Confidence.* 2010.

Newman, Jack. *The Ultimate Breastfeeding Book of Answers: The Most Comprehensive Problem-Solution Guide to Breastfeeding from the Foremost Expert in North America.* 2006.

Pantell, Robert H. and James F. Fries. *Taking Care of Your Child, Ninth Edition: A Parent's Illustrated Guide to Complete Medical Care.* 2015.

Peterson, Gayle. *Making Healthy Families.* 2000.

Satter, Ellyn. *Child of Mine: Feeding with Love and Good Sense.* 2000.

Simkin, Penny, April Bolding, Ann Keppler, Janelle Durham, and Janet Walley. *Pregnancy, Childbirth, and the Newborn: The Complete Guide.* 2015.

Sloan, Mark. *Birth Day: A Pediatrician Explores the Science, the History, and the Wonder of Childbirth.* 2014.

Spock, Benjamin and Robert Needlman. *Dr. Spock's Baby and Child Care.* 2011.

Magazines

American Baby
www.parents.com/american-baby-magazine
This magazine is for expectant and new parents; it covers baby issues from preconception to age two years.

Babytalk
www.parenting.com/Babytalk/babytalk.jsp?genID=7
This magazine offers articles, tips, and chats on raising your baby.

Consumer Reports
www.consumerreports.org
This magazine reviews baby products, and its accompanying website issues important information about safety standards and recalls.

Mothering
www.mothering.com
This magazine features philosophical inspiration and practical advice about natural family living.

Parenting
www.parenting.com
This magazine offers articles, tips, and chats on all topics concerning pregnancy and raising a child.

Parents
www.parents.com
This magazine is written to help parents raise healthy, happy families.

Working Mother
www.workingmother.com
This magazine is dedicated to the lives of working women and mothers.

Resource Groups

Low-Cost Care Resources

Child Welfare League of America
www.cwla.org
877-KIDS-NOW (877-543-7669)
This organization has information about low-cost medical care. Medicaid funds are available for pregnant women and children younger than six years old whose family income is less than a certain amount. Contact them to find the phone numbers for Medicaid agencies in your state. Your state agency can tell you whether you qualify for medical assistance.

Women, Infants, and Children (WIC)
www.fns.usda.gov/wic
The WIC program offers food for pregnant women and breastfeeding help for new mothers whose income is less than a certain amount. They can also help you find parenting help and support. Also, your care provider may help you find your local WIC office.

Pregnancy Resources

Baby-Friendly USA
www.babyfriendlyusa.org
This source provides a list of "baby-friendly" hospitals and birth centers that have policies to encourage breastfeeding.

Centers for Disease Control (CDC) on Pregnancy
www.cdc.gov/ncbddd/pregnancy_gateway /before.html
This CDC web page features tips for staying healthy before and during pregnancy.

Childbirth Connection
www.childbirthconnection.org
This nonprofit's website features a discussion of maternity care options.

International Cesarean Awareness Network (ICAN)
www.childbirth.org/section/ICAN.html
This organization has information for mothers about cesarean births and how to best recover from them.

March of Dimes
www.marchofdimes.com
March of Dimes seeks to prevent premature birth and birth defects. You can find helpful information about staying healthy during pregnancy, and preparing and caring for your baby on their website.

National Newborn Screening and Genetics Regulation Center (NNSGRC)
www.genes-r-us.uthscsa.edu
This resource can help you learn about specific newborn screenings and tests.

Baby Care Resources

American Academy of Pediatrics
www.aap.org
847-434-4000
This organization offers information about parenting, keeping your child healthy, and finding a pediatrician.

American SIDS Institute
www.sids.org
800-232-SIDS (800-232-7437)
This organization provides information about ways to reduce the risk of SIDS.

Automotive Safety Program
www.preventinjury.org
800-543-6227
If your child has special needs, she may need a car seat that's custom designed for her situation.

Centers for Disease Control (CDC) on Vaccination Safety
www.cdc.gov/vaccinesafety
This CDC web page has information on vaccination schedules and common concerns.

Child Care Aware
www.childcareaware.org
800-424-2246
Child Care Aware is a resource to find high-quality child care.

Consumer Product Safety Commission (CPSC)
www.cpsc.gov
301-504-7923
This agency offers information about home safety and unsafe baby-care products.

Environmental Protection Agency (EPA)
www.epa.gov
202-272-0167
This agency has helpful guidelines for making your home baby friendly.

Immunization Action Coalition
www.immunize.org
651-647-9009 (Hotline for questions about vaccines: 800-232-2522)
This organization offers information about vaccinations to keep your baby healthy.

Juvenile Products Manufacturers Association (JPMA)
www.jpma.org
This national trade organization is dedicated to the safe use of juvenile products. Use their website to find out whether baby gear has their safety certification.

KidsHealth
www.kidshealth.org
This website includes information for parents and kids about children's health and development. It features individual articles on such issues as developmental disabilities, medical problems, first aid, and nutrition.

National Highway Traffic Safety Administration (NHTSA)
www.nhtsa.gov
888-DASH-2-DOT (888-327-4236)
Their Child Passenger Safety (CPS) Department offers information about infant and child car seats.

National Association for the Education of Young Children (NAEYC)
www.naeyc.org
You can find day care guidelines and contact information here.

National Association of Child Care Resource and Referral Agencies
www.naccrra.org
This organization works with referral agencies to provide parents with safe child-care options.

National Vaccine Center
www.nvic.org
This organization provides parents with information on vaccine safety.

Safe Kids USA
www.safekids.org
This website provides safety guidelines for individual age groups and includes information on product recalls.

Seat Check
www.seatcheck.org
866-SEAT-CHECK
This national campaign to help parents properly secure their children in motor vehicles features a free child safety-seat inspection, available at their website or by calling their toll-free phone number.

SIDS Alliance (First Candle)
www.sidsalliance.org
800-221-7437
This organization provides information about sudden infant death syndrome (SIDS) and other causes of infant death. They offer suggestions about safe sleeping.

United States Agriculture Department
www.nutrition.gov
http://choosemyplate.gov
This agency's websites include information on nutrition, healthy eating, physical activity, and food safety.

Breastfeeding Resources

Human Milk Banking Association of North America (HMBANA)
www.hmbana.org
This association of milk banks carefully screens and pasteurizes donated breast milk before sending it out to mothers and babies in need.

International Lactation Consultant Association (ILCA)
www.ilca.org
This association keeps records of breastfeeding professionals who are International Board Certified Lactation Consultants (IBCLC). Contact them to find a breastfeeding expert in your area.

La Leche League (LLL)
www.lalecheleague.org
847-519-7730
This organization offers mother-baby groups for breastfeeding support. Contact them to find a LLL group near you. Or ask them to help you find breastfeeding consultants in your area.

Parenting Resources

County, State, or City Public Health Department
These departments can give you information about agencies that offer help with parenting issues. Contact the health department for your state, county, or city to learn more about parenting resources near you.

Attachment Parenting International (API)
www.attachmentparenting.org
API is a nonprofit organization that supports the philosophy of attachment parenting. Their website features links to support groups and literature.

Autism Speaks
www.autismspeaks.org
This autism advocacy group has a resource library and updated information for parents of children with autism.

Family Equality Council
www.familyequality.org
The Family Equality Council is a source for LGBTQ-headed families and the local groups that support them.

National Healthy Mothers, Healthy Babies Coalition
www.hmhb.org
703-836-6110
This organization offers help with breastfeeding and parenting.

National Information Center for Children and Youth with Disabilities (NICHCY)
www.nichcy.org
800-695-0285
This organization provides information on disabilities in children and youth; programs and services for infants, children, and youth with disabilities; and more.

National Organization of Mothers of Twins Clubs, Inc.
www.nomotc.org
877-540-2200
This organization provides information and support for families having more than one baby. Contact them to learn the names of local groups for parents of multiples.

Parents Anonymous, Inc.
www.parentsanonymous.org
909-621-6184
This organization works toward the prevention and treatment of child abuse. Treatment blends support groups with self-help.

Parents Without Partners
www.parentswithoutpartners.org
561-391-8833
This organization provides information and support for single parents and their children. Contact them to find a group in your area.

Planned Parenthood
www.plannedparenthood.org
800-230-PLAN (800-230-7526)
This organization provides reproductive health care, including birth control, as well as affordable medical care, including cancer screening.

Prevent Child Abuse America
www.preventchildabuse.org
877-224-8223
This volunteer-based coalition's goals are to foster awareness of the problem and to develop effective child abuse prevention programs.

MyChild
www.cerebralpalsy.org
This organization for parents of children with cerebral palsy includes information about medical care, financial assistance, and other important topics.

Your Local Community College
Many community colleges have classes for parents. Contact the family life education department at your local community college.

Postpartum Depression and Loss Resources

Postpartum Support International
www.postpartum.net
800-944-4773
This group offers help to women with postpartum mood disorders. Contact them to learn about a mothers' support group in your area.

Share Pregnancy & Infant Loss Support, Inc.
www.nationalshare.org
800-821-6819
This group offers support for families who have lost a baby by early pregnancy loss, stillbirth, or newborn death.

Solace for Mothers
www.solaceformothers.org
This organization provides help for mothers who have had a traumatic birth experience.

Online Support Groups

MotheringDotCommune
www.mothering.com/discussions

Parenting Forums
www.parentingforums.com

Birth to 24 months: Girls
Length-for-age and Weight-for-age percentiles

NAME _____

RECORD # _____

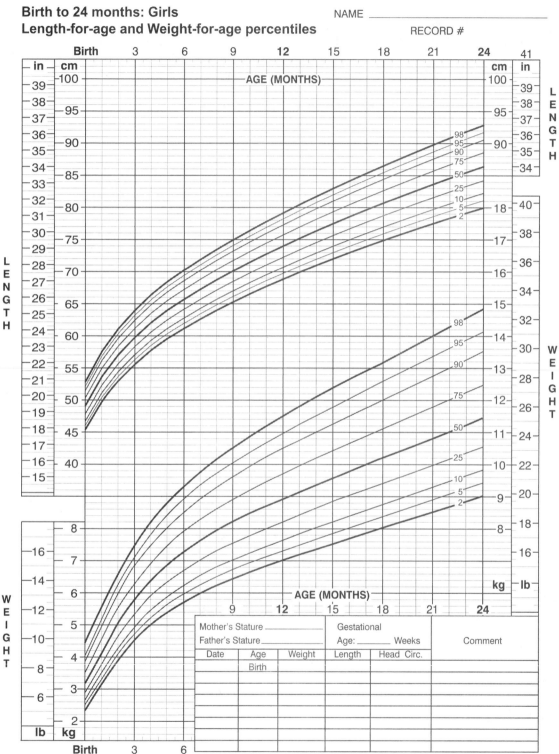

Published by the Centers for Disease Control and Prevention, November 1, 2009
SOURCE: WHO Child Growth Standards (http://www.who.int/childgrowth/en)

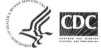

Birth to 24 months: Boys
Length-for-age and Weight-for-age percentiles

NAME _____

RECORD # _____

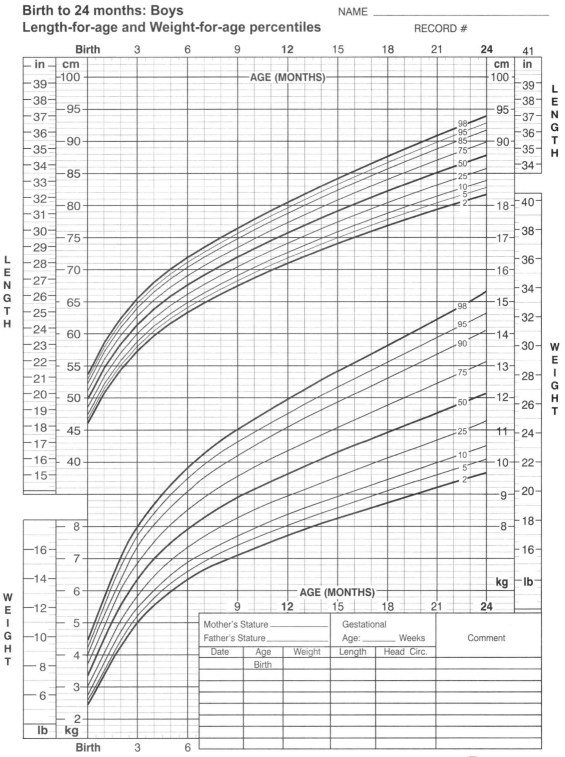

Index

Also from
Meadowbrook Press

Baby Play & Learn Child-development expert Penny Warner offers 160 ideas for games and activities that provide hours of developmental learning opportunities. It includes bulleted lists of skills baby learns through play, step-by-step instructions for each game and activity, and illustrations that demonstrate how to play many of the games.

Baby & Child Emergency First Aid edited by Mitchell J. Einzig, MD. This user-friendly book is the next best thing to 911, with a quick-reference index, large illustrations, and easy-to-read instructions on handling the most common childhood emergencies.

Feed Me! I'm Yours is an easy-to-use, economical guide to making baby food at home. More than 200 recipes cover everything a parent needs to know about teething foods, nutritious snacks, and quick, pleasing lunches.

The Toddler's Busy Book, *The Preschooler's Busy Book*, and *The Arts and Crafts Busy Book* each contains 365 activities (one for each day of the year) for your children, using items found around the home. The books offer parents and child-care providers fun reading, math, and science activities that will stimulate a child's natural curiosity. They also provide great activities for indoor play during even the longest stretches of bad weather!

Pregnancy, Childbirth, and the Newborn This book covers all aspects of childbearing, from conception through early infancy. It offers detailed information, suggestions, and advice to help make pregnancy, childbirth, and new parenthood an enjoyable, healthy experience. It presents the latest research-based information, including new information on complementary medicine approaches, updated information on interventions during childbirth, and new advice to help you make informed decisions about your care. It's the most authoritative, yet easy to use.
Extra information, resources, and worksheets are located on PCNGuide.com.

**We offer many more titles written to delight, inform, and entertain.
To browse our full selection of titles, visit our website at:**

www.MeadowbrookPress.com

For quantity discounts, please call: 1-800-338-2232

Meadowbrook Press